Endocrinology and Diabetes

CLINICAL CASES UNCOVERED

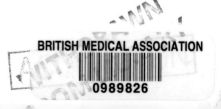

This book is dedicated to my daughter Nour and wife Manar, for their care, patience and support, and to my parents for their constant encouragement

Endocrinology and Diabetes

CLINICAL CASES UNCOVERED

Ramzi Ajjan

MRCP, MMed Sci, PhD

Senior Lecturer and Honorary Consultant
in Diabetes and Endocrinology
Department of Health Clinician Scientist
The LIGHT Laboratories
University of Leeds
Leeds, UK

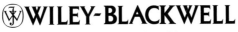

WILEY-BLACKWELL

A John Wiley & Sons, Ltd., Publication

This edition first published 2009, © 2009 by R. Ajjan

Blackwell Publishing was acquired by John Wiley & Sons in February 2007. Blackwell's publishing program has been merged with Wiley's global Scientific, Technical and Medical business to form Wiley-Blackwell.

Registered office: John Wiley & Sons Ltd, The Atrium, Southern Gate, Chichester, West Sussex, PO19 8SQ, UK

Editorial offices: 9600 Garsington Road, Oxford, OX4 2DQ, UK

The Atrium, Southern Gate, Chichester, West Sussex, PO19 8SQ, UK

111 River Street, Hoboken, NJ 07030-5774, USA

For details of our global editorial offices, for customer services and for information about how to apply for permission to reuse the copyright material in this book please see our website at www.wiley.com/wiley-blackwell

The right of the author to be identified as the author of this work has been asserted in accordance with the Copyright, Designs and Patents Act 1988.

Wiley also publishes its books in a variety of electronic formats. Some content that appears in print may not be available in electronic books.

Designations used by companies to distinguish their products are often claimed as trademarks. All brand names and product names used in this book are trade names, service marks, trademarks or registered trademarks of their respective owners. The publisher is not associated with any product or vendor mentioned in this book. This publication is designed to provide accurate and authoritative information in regard to the subject matter covered. It is sold on the understanding that the publisher is not engaged in rendering professional services. If professional advice or other expert assistance is required, the services of a competent professional should be sought.

Library of Congress Cataloging-in-Publication Data
Ajjan, Ramzi.
    Endocrinology and diabetes : clinical cases uncovered / Ramzi Ajjan.
        p. ; cm.
    Includes index.
    ISBN 978-1-4051-5726-1
    1. Endocrinology – Case studies. 2. Diabetes – Case studies.   I. Title.
    [DNLM: 1. Endocrine System Diseases – diagnosis – Case Reports.   2. Diabetes Mellitus –
diagnosis – Case Reports.   3. Diabetes Mellitus – therapy – Case Reports.   4. Endocrine System
Diseases – therapy – Case Reports.   WK 140 A312e 2009]
    RC649.5.A35 2009
    616.4 – dc22

                                                                                                        2008033368

ISBN: 978-1-4051-5726-1

A catalogue record for this book is available from the British Library.

Set in 9/12pt Minion by SNP Best-set Typesetter Ltd., Hong Kong
Printed and bound in Singapore by Fabulous Printers Pte Ltd

3   2012

Contents

(Part 3) Self-assessment, 164

Colour plate section can be found facing p. 84.

Preface

Almost two decades have passed since my medical student days and I still remember how difficult, and often tedious, it was to read and understand some of the clinical topics presented in textbooks.

Having been fortunate enough for my career to develop in academic medicine, part of my work involves regular teaching and lecturing at different levels, ranging from medical students to experienced physicians and health care professionals.

Despite a variety of audience, there has always been a general enthusiasm for further learning when clinical tutorials/lectures were not only presented as 'facts' but also as case-based studies. Moreover, I realised during my clinical practice that various medical conditions are best remembered by discussing and fully evaluating real life cases. Putting things together, I felt a case-based book would offer a unique opportunity to facilitate understanding of clinical diabetes and endocrinology, and make the learning process an enjoyable experience.

In Part 1 of the book, a simple reminder of clinical diabetes and endocrine conditions is provided, including basic science, symptoms and signs, investigations and treatment.

In Part 2, diabetes and endocrinology are covered using 'real life' cases, which I encountered during my clinical practice. Each case is divided into a number of sections/questions, which you should read carefully and make an attempt to give a differential diagnosis or formulate a management plan. You will notice I have varied the amount of background information, depending on the importance and the prevalence of the medical condition under discussion. In common clinical scenarios, comprehensive management plans are given, whereas in less common and more specialised cases, diagnostic and treatment strategies are only briefly touched upon. Take your time with each case and remember that these are real life cases, which you may be attending to as a junior medical doctor.

Ramzi Ajjan

Acknowledgements

My thanks and appreciation extend to a large number of individuals who contributed to this book by providing appropriate cases and different illustrations, including Dr Steve Orme, Dr Paul Belchetz, Dr Carol Amery, Dr Michael Waller, Dr Robert Bury, Mr Bernard Chang, Professor David Gawkrodger and Professor Steve Atkin. I am indebted to the Radiology and Radionuclide Departments at Leeds General Infirmary and I also wish to thank the Medical Photography Department for putting up with my repeated requests. I acknowledge the help of my Registrar, Dr Thet Koko, for sourcing appropriate illustrations. Special thanks go to my Secretary, Krystyna Pierzchalski for her patience and invaluable support.

Finally, I would like to thank Professor Anthony Weetman and Professor Peter Grant for their guidance over the years, which has been vital for my academic progress, and Dr Steve Orme for his unwavering support through my clinical career.

How to use this book

Clinical Cases Uncovered (CCU) books are carefully designed to help supplement your clinical experience and assist with refreshing your memory when revising. Each book is divided into three sections: Part 1, Basics; Part 2, Cases; and Part 3, Self-Assessment.

Part 1 gives a quick reminder of the basic science, history and examination, and key diagnoses in the area. Part 2 contains many of the clinical presentations you would expect to see on the wards or crop up in exams, with questions and answers leading you through each case. New information, such as test results, is revealed as events unfold and each case concludes with a handy case summary explaining the key points. Part 3 allows you to test your learning with several question styles (MCQs, EMQs and SAQs), each with a strong clinical focus.

Whether reading individually or working as part of a group, we hope you will enjoy using your CCU book. If you have any recommendations on how we could improve the series, please do let us know by contacting us at: medstudentuk@oxon.blackwellpublishing.com.

Disclaimer

CCU patients are designed to reflect real life, with their own reports of symptoms and concerns. Please note that all names used are entirely fictitious and any similarity to patients, alive or dead, is coincidental.

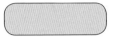 # List of abbreviations

ABG	arterial blood gas (analysis)	5HIAA	5-hydroxyindolacetic acid
ACEI	angiotensin converting enzyme inhibitors	HNF	hepatic nuclear factor
ACR	albumin/creatinine ratio	HMG	CoA 3-hydroxy, 3-methylglutaryl coenzyme A
ACTH	adrenocorticotrophic hormone	HONK	hyperosmolar non-ketotic hyperglycaemia
AD	autosomal dominant	HRT	hormone replacement therapy
ADH	antidiuretic hormone	IHD	ischaemic heart disease
AH	autoimmune hypothyroidism	IHH	idiopathic hypogonadotrophic hypogonadism
AP	alkaline phosphatase	IST	insulin stress test
AR	autosomal recessive	IUI	intrauterine insemination
ARB	angiotensin receptor blocker	i.v.	intravenous
BMD	bone mineral density	IVF	in vitro fertilization
BMI	body mass index	LADA	latent autoimmune diabetes of adults
CAH	congenital adrenal hyperplasia	LDLc	low-density lipoprotein cholesterol
CCF	congestive cardiac failure	LDST	low dose synacthen test
CRH	corticotrophin releasing hormone	LFT	liver function test
CRP	C-reactive protein	LH	luteinizing hormone
CT	computed tomography	MEN	multiple endocrine neoplasia
CVA	cerebrovascular accident	MIBG	meta-iodobenzylguanidine
DEXA	dual energy X-ray absorptiometry	MODY	maturity onset diabetes of the young
DHEA	dehydroepiandrosterone	MRA	magnetic resonance angiography
DI	diabetes insipidus	MRI	magnetic resonance imaging
DKA	diabetic ketoacidosis	MTC	medullary thyroid cancer
DOC	deoxycorticosterone	NF	neurofibromatosis
DPP	dipeptidyl peptidase	OCP	oral contraceptive pill
ECG	electrocardiogram	OGT	oral glucose tolerance (test)
ESR	erythrocyte sedimentation rate	PCOS	polycystic ovary syndrome
FBC	full blood count	PE	pulmonary embolus
FHH	familial hypocalciuric hypercalcaemia	PRA	plasma renin activity
FNA	fine needle aspiration	PRL	prolactin
FSH	follicle stimulating hormone	PSA	prostate specific antigen
GAD	glutamic acid decarboxylase	PTH	parathyroid hormone
GGT	gamma glutamyl transpeptidase	RAI	radioactive iodine
GH	growth hormone	SHBG	sex hormone binding globulin
GHRH	growth hormone releasing hormone	SIADH	syndrome of inappropriate ADH secretion
GLP	glucagon-like peptide	TC	total cholesterol
GnRH	gonadotrophin releasing hormone	T1DM	type 1 diabetes mellitus
GO	Graves' ophthalmopathy	T2DM	type 2 diabetes mellitus
GST	glucagon stimulation test	TFT	thyroid function test
hCG	human chorionic gonadotrophin	TG	thyroglobulin

TIA	transient ischaemic attack	TSH	thyroid stimulating hormone (thyrotropin)
TMNG	toxic multinodular goitre	U&Es	urea and electrolytes
TN	toxic solitary nodule	UTI	urinary tract infection
TPO	thyroid peroxidase	VIP	vasoactive intestinal peptide
TRH	thyrotropin releasing hormone		

The pituitary gland

Understanding the pituitary gland is probably the hardest part of endocrinology as it controls most of the endocrine glands in the body and disease may arise due to both over-secretion and undersecretion of a particular hormone. A full understanding of the hormonal tests in this section will make interpretation of the endocrine tests in the rest of the book an easy and pleasant experience.

Anatomy

The pituitary gland is situated in the pituitary fossa and is surrounded by (see Fig. 1):
- Below: sphenoid air sinus
- Either side: cavernous sinus and carotid artery
- Above: the pituitary stalk extending into the hypothalamus

Physiology

The pituitary gland can be functionally divided into two lobes (Fig. 2)
- The anterior pituitary, which *produces* the following hormones
  - Growth hormone (GH): resulting in skeletal growth
  - Adrenocorticotrophic hormone (ACTH): stimulates the adrenals to produce steroids
  - Gonadotrophins (FSH and LH): stimulate the testicles or ovaries to produce sex hormones
  - Thyroid stimulating hormone or thyrotrophin (TSH): stimulates the thyroid to produce thyroid hormones
  - Prolactin (PRL): stimulates breast milk production
- The posterior pituitary, which *stores* the hormones produced in the hypothalamus (does not produce them)

Endocrinology and Diabetes: Clinical Cases Uncovered. By R. Ajjan. Published 2009 by Blackwell Publishing, ISBN: 978-1-4051-5726-1

  - Antidiuretic hormone (ADH): stimulates water reabsorption by the kidneys
  - Oxytocin: helps uterine contractions during labour

The anterior pituitary gland is under the control of the hypothalamus as shown in Fig. 3.
- Corticotrophin releasing hormone (CRH): stimulates ACTH secretion
- Growth hormone releasing hormone (GHRH): stimulates GH secretion
- Thyrotrophin releasing hormone (TRH): stimulates TSH secretion
- Gonadotrophin releasing hormone (GnRH): stimulates FSH and LH secretion
- Prolactin releasing hormone does not exist and prolactin is under the inhibitory effect of the hypothalamus

Cortisol, GH, thyroid hormones and sex hormones all have a negative feedback effect on corresponding pituitary (ACTH, GH, TSH and FSH/LH respectively) and hypothalamic (CRH, GHRH, TRH and GnRH respectively) hormone release.

Clinical disease

Clinical disease results from oversecretion or undersecretion of pituitary hormones, in addition to the local compressive effects of a pituitary tumour. A pituitary tumour may secrete excessive hormones but it may also be non-functional, in which case the clinical presentation consists of pituitary failure associated with compressive effects.

Pituitary oversecretion
- Usually due to pituitary tumours overproducing one hormone (sometimes more than one) resulting in typical clinical entities, which are described below
- Very rarely, overproduction of pituitary hormones may be due to increased production of pituitary hormone releasing hormones (CRH, GHRH)

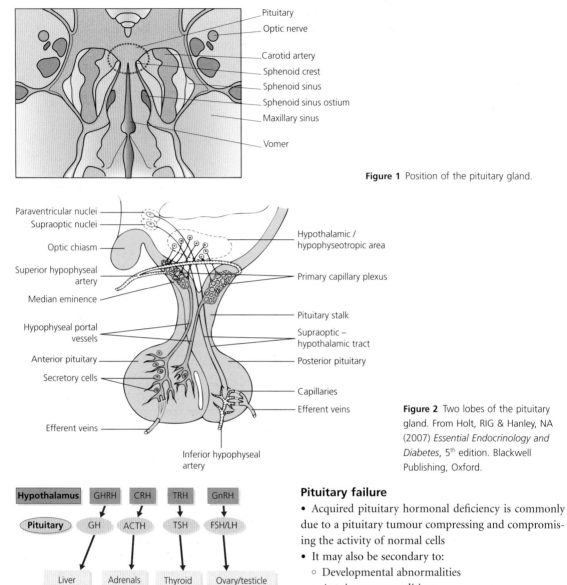

Figure 1 Position of the pituitary gland.

Figure 2 Two lobes of the pituitary gland. From Holt, RIG & Hanley, NA (2007) *Essential Endocrinology and Diabetes*, 5th edition. Blackwell Publishing, Oxford.

Figure 3 Control of hormone secretion by the hypothalamus and pituitary (see text). GHRH, CRH, TRH and GnRH, secreted by the hypothalamus, stimulate GH, ACTH, TSH and FSH/LH production by the pituitary respectively, which in turn stimulate the liver, adrenal glands, thyroid and ovaries/testicles to produce their hormones. GH, adrenal steroids, thyroid hormones and sex steroids in turn have a negative feedback effect (reduce hormone production) on the corresponding hypothalamic/pituitary hormone release. The pituitary hormone prolactin (which is not shown here) is unique as there is no hypothalamic hormone to stimulate its release but it is rather under inhibitory control.

Pituitary failure

- Acquired pituitary hormonal deficiency is commonly due to a pituitary tumour compressing and compromising the activity of normal cells
- It may also be secondary to:
  - Developmental abnormalities
  - Autoimmune conditions
  - Head injury
  - Vascular disorders and severe blood loss (resulting in infarction of the pituitary)
  - Infiltrative disease and infection (sarcoidosis, tuberculosis)
  - Radiotherapy
- It should be noted that pituitary hormonal deficiency commonly involves multiple hormones and, therefore, deficiency of one hormone warrants full pituitary investigations.
- Local effects of all pituitary tumours include:
  - Headaches

○ Visual field defects (usually bitemporal hemianopia)
○ Deficiency of other hormones (due to pressure effect on normal pituitary tissue)
○ Cranial nerve palsies: 3rd, 4th and 6th in large pituitary tumours

Investigations of the pituitary gland

This involves investigations of hormonal abnormalities and imaging of the pituitary gland.

Hormonal investigation of suspected pituitary hormone abnormality

In general, there are three ways to investigate hormonal abnormalities in endocrine disease:

* Static hormone measurements: this is a "one off" measurement of a particular hormone. Examples include measurement of thyroid function (TSH and T4), gonadal function (sex steroids and gonadotrophins) and measurement of prolactin
* Stimulation tests: if deficiency of a particular hormone is suspected, stimulation tests are carried out. Failure of a particular hormone level to rise after stimulation tests confirms hormonal deficiency. Examples include growth hormone and cortisol deficiency
* Suppression test: if oversecretion of a hormone is suspected, suppression tests can be carried out. Failure of suppression of a particular hormone indicates overproduction. Examples include growth hormone oversecretion (acromegaly) and ACTH oversecretion (Cushing's disease)

Static pituitary function tests
Thyroid function tests (TFTs)
* Low free T4 (FT4) with low or low normal TSH:
  ○ This should alert to the possibility of pituitary failure
  ○ Differential diagnosis includes abnormal TFTs due to non-thyroidal illness (described in the thyroid section)
* Raised TSH and raised FT4: possible TSH-secreting pituitary tumour
* Raised TSH with low or normal FT4: primary hypothyroidism
* Suppressed TSH with high or normal FT4: primary hyperthyroidism
Sex hormones (testosterone or oestradiol)
* Low sex hormones with low or low normal gonadotrophins (FSH and LH) should raise the possibility of pituitary failure

* High sex steroids with elevated gonadotrophin suggest gonadotrophin-secreting pituitary tumour (these are rare and often clinically silent)
* Low sex hormones with raised gonadotrophins, indicate primary gonadal failure and this is seen in physiological menopause (women above the age of 50 usually have raised gonadotrophin levels with low oestradiol)
Prolactin
* Raised serum prolactin may be due to a pituitary prolactinoma (this is fully discussed later in this chapter)

Stimulation tests in suspected hypopituitarism
The two main stimulation tests used are:

Insulin stress test
* This is the gold standard test to assess pituitary function but it has a number of contraindications (see below) and therefore it is not always used first line
* Insulin injection results in hypoglycaemia creating a stressful environment with consequent release of ACTH and GH
* 0.1–0.3 U/kg of insulin is injected (high doses are required in those with insulin resistance) to render the patient hypoglycaemic and GH/cortisol are measured
* GH >20 mIU/L and cortisol >580 nmol/L indicate adequate hormonal reserve
* Contraindications
  ○ History of epilepsy
  ○ Abnormal ECG or ischemic heart disease
  ○ Untreated hypothyroidism
  ○ Basal cortisol < 100 nmol/L

Glucagon stimulation test
* Injection of glucagon results in:
  ○ Release of growth hormone and ACTH (GH >20 mIU/L or cortisol >580 nmol/L indicate normal GH and ACTH reserve)
* The test is not always reliable (up to 20% of normal individuals fail to fully respond) and in case of any doubts insulin stress test should be performed
* Contraindications
  ○ The test is less reliable in subjects with diabetes

Other stimulation tests
* These are quite specialized and beyond the scope of this book and include:
  ○ TRH stimulation test
  ○ GnRH stimulation test
  ○ Arginine stimulation test

Table 1 Main tests for pituitary functions.

Static tests	Stimulation tests	Suppression tests
Thyroid function tests Low FT4 and low or low-normal TSH suggests hypopituitarism	**Insulin stress test** Failure of GH and cortisol to rise after insulin injection suggests hypopituitarism	**Glucose tolerance test** Failure of GH suppression after oral GTT suggests GH oversecretion (acromegaly)
Sex hormones Low sex hormones with low or low-normal gonadotrophins suggests hypopituitarism	**Glucagon stimulation tests** Failure of GH and cortisol to rise after glucagon injection suggests hypopituitarism	**Low- and high-dose dexamethasone suppression test** (see text)
Prolactin Raised prolactin suggests pituitary prolactinoma		

Suppression tests in suspected hormonal overproduction
Oral glucose tolerance test
- This is used in suspected GH oversecretion
  - Failure to suppress GH to <2 mIU/L after 75 g oral glucose tolerance test strongly suggests the diagnosis of acromegaly

Dexamethasone suppression test
- This is used to diagnose Cushing's syndrome but may also be able to differentiate between pituitary and non-pituitary causes of Cushing's syndrome
  - Low dose dexamethasone suppression test: failure to suppress cortisol to <50 nmol/L after giving 0.5 mg of dexamethasone 6 hourly for 2 days, suggests the diagnosis of Cushing's syndrome
  - Suppression of cortisol to >50% of basal levels after giving 2 mg of dexamethasone 6 hourly for 2 days suggest pituitary cause (i.e. Cushing's disease)
  The main tests for pituitary function are summarized in Table 1.

Imaging of the pituitary gland
Magnetic resonance imaging (MRI)
- This is the gold standard for imaging of the pituitary gland (Fig. 4 shows a pituitary adenoma that enhances after godalinium injection)

Combination of imaging with stimulation tests
- In some complicated cases it may be necessary to perform inferior petrosal sinus sampling under radiological guidance followed by stimulation tests

- High levels of pituitary hormones in the petrosal sinus compared with a peripheral vein, confirm the diagnosis of pituitary secreting hormones
  - The test is often used to differentiate pituitary-dependent Cushing's disease from ectopic ACTH secretion. Higher ACTH levels in the petrosal sinus compared with venous ACTH, after CRH stimulation confirms pituitary-dependent Cushing's disease

Treatment
- Non-functioning pituitary tumours or those associated with increased hormone production (except for prolactinomas, see below) are usually treated surgically:
  - Transphenoidal surgery (in most cases)
  - Transcranial surgery (rarely, in very large tumours)
- Pituitary hormone deficiency should be treated by hormone replacement (pituitary failure is usually associated with multiple hormonal deficiencies)

Clinical disease of the anterior pituitary gland
This section discusses the effects of over- and underproduction of a particular hormone.

Abnormalities of growth hormone secretion
Growth hormone excess
In childhood or adolescence growth hormone excess results in:
- Excessive growth spurt
- Increased size of feet and hands
- General skeletal enlargement
- Increased skin thickness

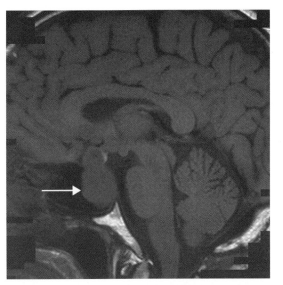

(a)

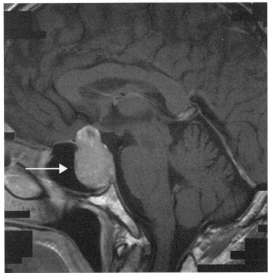

(b)

Figure 4 MRI of the pituitary showing a pituitary adenoma, before (a) and after (b) gadolinium injection.

• If left untreated, growth hormone excess in this period of life leads to gigantism, the most serious consequence of the disease

In adults, growth hormone excess affects the skin, soft tissue and skeleton resulting in acromegaly, which has the following features:

• Acromegalic face (coarse facial features, see Fig. 5, colour plate section)
  ○ Prominent supraorbital ridges
  ○ Large nose
  ○ Lower jaw pushed forward (prognathism)
  ○ Thickening of lips and tongue
  ○ Dental malocclusion and widely spaced teeth
• Wide and large hands/feet (enlargement of soft tissue, skin and cartilage), typically presenting with
  ○ Increasing glove size
  ○ Tight-fitting rings
  ○ Increasing shoe size
• Deep voice
• Nerve entrapment: carpal tunnel syndrome is not uncommon (soft tissue enlargement)
• Increased sweating (common complaint)
• Organomegaly
  ○ Goitre
  ○ Cardiomegaly
  ○ Hepatomegaly
  ○ Splenomegaly
• Complications of acromegaly include (may be the presenting feature of the disease):
  ○ Hypertension
  ○ Diabetes
  ○ Obstructive sleep apnoea
  ○ Increased risk of heart disease
  ○ Increased risk of colonic polyps and colonic carcinoma

Investigations
• Random GH
  ○ A random GH of <1 mIU/L makes the diagnosis of acromegaly unlikely
  ○ A random GH >1 mIU/L does not help in making a diagnosis
• Glucose tolerance test
  ○ Failure of GH suppression after GTT suggests the diagnosis of acromegaly
• Insulin-like growth factor-1 (IGF-1) levels
  ○ These are elevated in acromegaly but this is mainly used to monitor response to therapy
• Imaging
  ○ Pituitary MRI: this usually shows a pituitary tumour

Treatment
• Transphenoidal surgery: the treatment of choice
• Radiotherapy: in patients with failed surgery or if surgery is contraindicated
• Medical treatment
  ○ Somatostatin analogues: used in patients with residual tumour post surgery or in whom surgery is contraindicated. It is effective at reducing GH levels in around 60% of patients

○ Dopamine agonists (cabergoline, bromocriptine): effective in a minority of patients

○ Pegvisomant: relatively new and effective treatment that blocks the growth hormone receptor but has no effect on growth hormone levels. The effect of this treatment on tumour size remains controversial

• Monitoring response to treatment

○ GH day curve: mean GH <5 mIU/L defines cure from the disease

○ IGF-1 levels: the aim is to normalize IGF-1 levels

○ Due to increased risk of colonic cancer, acromegaly patients should undergo regular colonoscopy for early detection of the disease

Growth hormone deficiency

In childhood, growth hormone deficiency (GHD) results in:

• Failure of growth

• Thin skin

• Hypoglycaemia (particularly in the presence of ACTH deficiency)

• Delayed puberty (particularly in the presence of sex hormone deficiency)

In adults, GHD results in non-specific symptoms:

• Tiredness

• Depression

• Reduction in muscle and increase in fat mass

The main clinical features of growth hormone excess/deficiency are summarized in Table 2.

Investigations

• Glucagon stimulation test or insulin stress tests

○ Failure of GH to rise after these stimulation tests suggests GHD

• IGF-1 levels

○ Low IGF-1 aids in the diagnosis. However, normal IGF-1 levels do not rule out the possibility of GHD

• Imaging

○ Pituitary MRI should be performed in subjects with GHD to rule out the possibility of pituitary tumour causing GHD by compressing GH-producing cells

Treatment

• Childhood GHD

○ GH replacement is necessary

• Adult GHD

○ Only symptomatic patients are usually offered GH replacement therapy

Table 2 Main symptoms, signs and complications of growth hormone excess and deficiency.

Growth hormone excess	Growth hormone deficiency
Symptoms	**Symptoms**
Fast growth (in children)	Failure of growth (in children)
Headaches (independent of local tumour effect)	Tiredness
	Depression
Increased sweating	Decreased body mass
Musculoskeletal pains	
Change in glove/ring and shoe size	
Signs	**Signs**
Facial appearance (see text)	Failure of growth and thin skin in children
Soft tissue and skeletal changes	No specific signs in adults
Organomegaly	
Visual field defect	
Deficiency of other pituitary hormones	
Complications	**Complications**
Hypertension	Short stature in untreated children
Diabetes	
Colonic polyps and colonic carcinoma	Hypoglycaemia (mainly in children)
Obstructive sleep apnoea	Osteoporosis in adults

Abnormalities of ACTH secretion
ACTH excess

Pituitary tumours producing ACTH result in excessive cortisol production by the adrenals, consequently leading to pituitary-dependent Cushing's syndrome (or Cushing's disease), which must be differentiated from other causes of Cushing's syndrome, including:

• Ectopic ACTH syndrome: due to the presence of malignant cells producing ACTH (lung cancer for example)

• Adrenal tumours: excess cortisol production is associated with suppression of ACTH production and, therefore, these tumours are usually referred to as non-ACTH dependent Cushing's syndrome

• Pseudo-Cushing's: excessive alcohol consumption or severe depression can result in symptoms and signs similar to Cushing's syndrome, and differentiating this from "real" Cushing's can sometimes be difficult even for an experienced endocrinologist

---

Box 1 Clinical features of Cushing's syndrome

- Growth arrest in children
- Typical facial appearance (see Fig. 6)
  - Round (moon-like) face
  - Acne
  - Hirsutism
  - Thinning of scalp hair
- Fat redistribution
  - Truncal obesity
  - Thin extremities
  - Supraclavicular fat pads
- Skin abnormalities
  - Thin skin
  - Striae on abdomen, breast and axillae (due to central obesity and thinning of the skin)
- Mood problems
  - Depression
  - Psychosis
  - Insomnia
- Sexual dysfunction
  - Low libido and impotence
  - Menstrual problems
- Complications
  - Hypertension
  - Diabetes mellitus
  - Osteoporosis
  - High risk of infections
  - Poor wound healing

Investigations

- Confirm the presence of excess cortisol
  - 24-hour urinary cortisol: high levels are suggestive of Cushing's syndrome
  - Midnight cortisol: in normal individuals, cortisol levels at midnight during sleep are undetectable. This test may be difficult to arrange as the patient needs to be admitted and a blood sample should be taken immediately after the patient is woken up
  - Overnight dexamethasone suppression test: give 0.5–1.0 mg of dexamethasone at 23:00 and measure cortisol at 09:00. Cortisol levels less than 50 nmol/L effectively rule out the diagnosis of Cushing's syndrome
  - Low dose dexamethasone suppression test: give 0.5 mg dexamethasone ever 6 hours for 2 days (eight

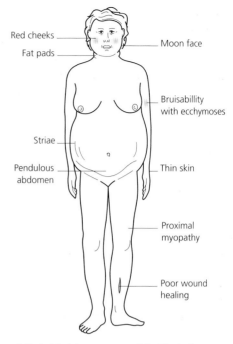

Figure 6 Typical facial appearance of Cushing's disease.

doses) and check cortisol levels thereafter, which should be undetectable in the absence of Cushing's syndrome
- Differentiate between different causes of Cushing's syndrome
  - ACTH levels: these are suppressed in adrenal Cushing's but detectable in pituitary Cushing's disease or cases due to ectopic ACTH production
  - High dose dexamethasone suppression test: give 2 mg dexamethasone every 6 h for 2 days. If cortisol is suppressed to more than 50% of basal value, it suggests a diagnosis of pituitary Cushing's disease
- Imaging
  - MRI of the pituitary: may show a pituitary tumour but it can sometimes be normal (tumour too small to visualize)
  - Petrosal sinus sampling: this may need to be undertaken in difficult cases to differentiate ectopic ACTH secretion from pituitary-dependent Cushing's disease

Treatment of Cushing's disease

- Transphenoidal surgery to remove the pituitary tumour

• Radiotherapy: in relapsed disease or in those whom surgery is contraindicated
• Adrenalectomy: in difficult cases (to stop cortisol secretion), but this is rarely performed

ACTH deficiency

This results in the failure of cortisol production by the adrenal glands. This results in:
• Failure of growth in children
• Malaise and tiredness
• Weight loss
• Hypoglycaemia
• Hypotension
• Confusion

The main clinical features of ACTH excess/deficiency are summarized in Table 3.

Investigations

• Pituitary stimulation tests (insulin stress test or glucagons stimulation test) fail to show adequate rise in serum cortisol levels
• The possibility of primary hypoadrenalism should be ruled out, in which case there is:
  ○ Low cortisol
  ○ High ACTH
• ACTH deficiency is usually part of panhypopituitarism and, therefore, deficiency of other hormones should be investigated
• In subjects with pure ACTH deficiency a CRH test may be necessary to confirm the diagnosis (failure of ACTH and cortisol to rise confirm ACTH deficiency)
• Imaging
  ○ Pituitary MRI to investigate the possibility of pituitary tumour

Treatment

• Cortisol replacement is necessary and usually oral hydrocortisone is used in two to three divided doses

Abnormalities of prolactin secretion
Prolactin excess

• Prolactinomas are the commonest functioning pituitary tumours
• Microprolactinomas are detected in up to 10% of the population in post-mortem studies
• Serum prolactin concentration may be elevated due to a large number of factors (summarized in Table 4), which should be differentiated from a prolactinoma.

Table 3 Main symptoms, signs and complications of ACTH excess and deficiency.

ACTH excess	ACTH deficiency
Symptoms	**Symptoms**
Failure of growth (in children)	Failure of growth (in children)
Weight gain	General malaise and weakness
Thin skin and easy bruising	Dizziness
Muscle weakness	Generalized aches and pains
Mood disturbances	Abdominal pain, diarrhoea and vomiting
Reduced libido and menstrual irregularities	Reduced libido and menstrual irregularities
Signs	**Signs**
Facial appearance (see text)	Postural hypotension
Truncal obesity, buffalo hump	Decreased axillary and pubic hair
Thin and fragile skin	
Abdominal and axillary striae	
Increased pigmentation due to high ACTH (skin and mucous membranes)	
Proximal muscle weakness	
Visual field defect	
Deficiency of other pituitary hormones	
Complications	**Complications**
Hypertension	Hypoglycaemia
Diabetes	Death
Osteoporosis	
Infections	

• Causes of raised plasma prolactin concentration seem to be a popular question in postgraduate medical examinations

Clinical presentation

Prolactinomas result in:
• Galactorrhoea (90% of women and 15% of men)
• Sexual dysfunction
• Decreased libido
• Menstrual irregularities
• Local tumour effects

Table 4 Causes of high plasma prolactin levels.

Physiological	Pregnancy
	Nipple stimulation
	Sexual intercourse
	Stress (simple venepuncture may cause PRL elevation)
Pituitary tumours	Prolactinoma
	Non-functioning tumours (elevation of prolactin is usually modest due to stalk compression and lack of inhibition of prolactin secretion)
Drugs	Large list including:
	Anti-emetics
	Antidepressants and antipsychotics
	Opiates
	Anti-HIV treatment
Hypothalamic disease	Tumours compressing the hypothalamus
	Infiltrative disease (sarcoidosis)
	Large pituitary tumours causing stalk compression
Metabolic	Hypothyroidism
	Chronic renal disease

Investigations
- Raised serum prolactin is suggestive of the diagnosis, provided other causes for raised prolactin are ruled out (see Table 4)
- Imaging
  - MRI of the pituitary usually shows a pituitary tumour, particularly in those with very high prolactin levels
  - In some patients no tumour can be identified but this does not rule out the diagnosis of prolactinoma (tumour can be too small)
  - In patients with a large pituitary tumour and only mild elevation of prolactin, a non-functioning pituitary adenoma rather than a prolactinoma should be suspected (raised prolactin in this case is due to stalk compression and 'escape' from the inhibitory effects of hypothalamus)

Treatment
- Pituitary prolactinomas are usually treated medically with dopamine agonists (cabergoline or bromocriptine), which result in both reduced hormone secretion and shrinkage of the tumour
- Surgery is reserved for severe cases that are not responding to medical treatment (and these are fortunately rare)
- It should be noted that prolactinomas are the only pituitary tumours where medical therapy, rather than surgery, is first-line treatment and, therefore, it is important to make the correct diagnosis in these cases

Prolactin deficiency
- Deficiency of prolactin results in failure of lactation in women with no other systemic effects
- This is usually part of other pituitary hormonal deficiency
- Can result from severe blood loss during childbirth, resulting in pituitary infarction, which is called Sheehan's syndrome
- There is no prolactin replacement therapy and deficiency of this hormone is not treated

Abnormalities in TSH secretion
TSH excess
TSH excess is rare and is usually due to a pituitary tumour (TSH-oma). It results in:
- Features of hyperthyroidism (clinical presentation is discussed in the chapter on the thyroid)
- Mass effect of the pituitary tumour (particularly as these tumours tend to be large)

Investigations
- High FT4 with high or normal TSH in subjects not on thyroxine replacement is suggestive of TSH-producing pituitary tumour
- Imaging
  - MRI of the pituitary: this usually shows a large tumour

Treatment
- Transphenoidal surgery
- Somatostatin analogues for recurrent or incompletely removed tumours
- Radiotherapy in case of recurrent tumour or unsuccessful surgery

TSH deficiency

TSH deficiency causes hypothyroidism (usually associated with other pituitary hormone deficiency).

The clinical features of hypothyroidism are discussed in the chapter on the thyroid.

Investigations

Low FT4 with low or normal TSH is suggestive of TSH deficiency and the pituitary gland should be fully evaluated for deficiencies of other pituitary hormones.

Treatment

• Thyroid hormone replacement in the form of synthetic T4 (levothyroxine)
• It should be noted that TSH measurements cannot be relied upon for monitoring the thyroxine dose, which is simply done by measuring FT4 levels and assessing the patient clinically
• In patients with combined ACTH and TSH deficiency, cortisol therapy should be started first and thryoxine replacement introduced a few days later to avoid precipitating an adrenal crisis

Abnormalities of gonadotrophin secretion
Gonadotrophin excess

Tumours producing FSH or LH are extremely rare and usually behave similarly to a non-functioning pituitary tumour. In men, FSH-secreting tumours may result in testicular enlargement.

Gonadotrophin deficiency

This results in sex hormone deficiency.

Clinical presentation

• Decreased libido, impotence and menstrual irregularities
• Loss of secondary sexual hair
• Loss of muscle mass in men
• In children
  ○ Delayed puberty and sexual infantilism
  ○ Primary amenorrhoea

Investigations

• Low testosterone in men and oestradiol in women with low or normal gonadotrophin levels, suggest secondary gonadal failure
• Imaging
  ○ Pituitary MRI should be performed in subjects with secondary gonadal failure

Treatment

• Treat the underlying cause
• Sex hormone replacement
  ○ Testosterone
  ○ Oestrogen and progesterone

Non-functioning pituitary adenoma

These are the commonest of pituitary macroadenomas. They present clinically with:
• Mass effect
• Visual field defect
• Headaches
• Cranial nerve palsies
• Hypopituitarism: resulting in GH, ACTH, TSH and gonadotrophin deficiencies (variable degrees), with the clinical manifestations described above

Investigations
Static pituitary function tests

• TFTs
• Sex hormones and gonadotrophin levels
• Prolactin (may be mildly elevated in non-functioning tumours; see section on prolactinoma)

Stimulation tests

• Insulin stress test or glucagon stimulation test to assess:
  ○ Cortisol (ACTH) reserve
  ○ GH reserve
• Suppression tests: only if there is a clinical suspicion of:

Box 2 Pituitary tumours

Pituitary tumours may be:
• Functional, secreting one or more hormones resulting in:
  ○ Galactorrhoea (prolactin)
  ○ Acromegaly (GH)
  ○ Cushing's syndrome (ACTH)
  ○ Hyperthyroidism (TSH)
• Non-functional, causing:
  ○ Mass effect
  ○ Anterior pituitary failure: this can be partial (one or two hormones) or total (involving all pituitary hormones)

Suspected pituitary tumours should be investigated with hormonal tests (rule out hyper- and hyposecretion of hormones) as well as imaging tests

- Cushing's syndrome
- Acromegaly
- Imaging
  - Pituitary MRI: shows a pituitary macroadenoma

Treatment

- Surgery: usually transphenoidal but transcranial surgery may be needed for larger tumours
- Radiotherapy: for recurrence
- Hormone replacement therapy: these patients usually end up with a mixture of pituitary hormonal deficiencies, which should be replaced

---

Box 3 Other causes of pituitary failure

- Pituitary infarction, characterized by:
  - Sudden onset headache
  - Cranial nerve palsies
  - Symptoms and signs of cortisol deficiency
- Pituitary infiltration
  - Sarcoidosis
  - Haemochromatosis
- Trauma
- Pituitary infection
  - Abscess
  - Tuberculosis
- Head irradiation
- Unknown causes
  Treatment of pituitary failure includes one or a cocktail of hormone replacement therapies:
- Steroids (hydrocortisone): anyone with suspected pituitary failure should be given hydrocortisone and investigated later (failure to give hydrocortisone in suspected deficiency may result in death)
- Thyroxine: should only be given after adequate cortisol replacement
- Testosterone (males), oestrogen and progesterone (females)
- Growth hormone: this is routinely given to children with GH deficiency but in adults, only those with symptoms receive this expensive form of treatment

---

The posterior pituitary

In contrast to the anterior pituitary, the posterior pituitary does not synthesize hormones but stores hormones produced in the hypothalamic region. These hormones include:
- Antidiuretic hormone (ADH)
- Oxytocin

Table 5 Causes of syndrome of inappropriate ADH (SIADH) secretion.

Tumours	Cancers: Lung malignancy, haematological malignancies, etc.
Central nervous system abnormalities	Infection (meningitis, encephalitis)
	Head injury
	Vascular disorders
Respiratory abnormalities	Infections
	Positive pressure ventilation
Drugs	Chemotherapy
	Anti-epileptic (carbamazepine)
	Oral hypoglycaemic (chlorpropamide)
	Antipsychotics
Endocrine	Hypothyroidism
Metabolic	Acute intermittent porphyria
Idiopathic	All above causes need ruling out before making this diagnosis

Abnormalities of ADH secretion

- Arginine-vasopressin or antidiuretic hormone
  - This hormone is secreted secondary to osmotic changes
  - Mediates free water reabsorption in the kidneys

Excessive ADH secretion – syndrome of inappropriate ADH secretion (SIADH)

This is not uncommonly seen on the medical wards and results in:
- Dilutional hyponatraemia
- Low plasma osmolarity and inappropriately high urine osmolarity (secondary to water reabsorption in the kidneys)
- Causes of inappropriate ADH secretion (known as syndrome of inappropriate ADH or SIADH) are summarized in Table 5.

Investigations

- Hyponatraemia is commonly seen in hospitalized patients. A common 'knee jerk reaction' is to label these patients as having SIADH and start fluid restriction, which can be detrimental if the patient is not assessed properly

• It should be remembered that patients with SIADH are euvolemic and therefore:
  ○ It is important to rule out dehydration before starting investigations for SIADH (are they on diuretics? is there a history of recent fluid loss?)
  ○ It is also important to rule out fluid overload before starting investigations for SIADH (is there advanced heart, liver or renal failure?)
• In euvolemic patients, SIADH should be suspected in the presence of:
  ○ Hyponatraemia with low plasma osmolarity
  ○ Inappropriately high urine osmolarity
  ○ High urinary sodium excretion
• In patients with suspected SIADH, we need to exclude:
  ○ Hypothyroidism (TFTs)
  ○ Hypoadrenalism (short synacthen test)
• Once the diagnosis of SIADH is made, it is necessary to establish the cause (see Table 5)
  ○ Careful history and examination of the patient
  ○ Double check drug history
  ○ Computed tomography (CT) head, chest and abdomen are frequently requested to rule out a malignant cause

Treatment
In confirmed SIADH:
• Restrict oral fluid to 750–1500 mL of oral fluid/day
• Treat the cause
• Demeclocycline, which induces nephrogenic diabetes insipidus, can help in difficult cases

ADH deficiency
This results in the passage of large volume of dilute urine, resulting in:
• Polyuria
• Nocturia
• Thirst
• Enuresis in children

Causes of ADH deficiency, also known as cranial diabetes insipidus (DI) are:
• Congenital or familial
• Acquired
  ○ Head injury
  ○ Tumours infiltrating the posterior pituitary
  ○ Infiltrative conditions, such as sarcoidosis or histiocytosis
  ○ Infections such as meningitis, encephalitis or tuberculosis
  ○ Vascular
  ○ Idiopathic

Functional ADH deficiency may occur if the kidneys fail to respond to the hormone (ADH production is normal). This is called nephrogenic DI, which may be:
• Congenital or familial
• Acquired
  ○ Drugs (lithium or demeclocycline)
  ○ Electrolyte abnormalities: hypercalcaemia, hypokalaemia
  ○ Chronic renal disease

Box 4 Abnormalities of oxytocin secretion

In women, oxytocin:
• Helps contraction of the pregnant uterus
• Helps contraction of breast duct smooth muscle aiding breast feeding
• Deficiency of this hormone has no effect on parturition or breast feeding
In men, the role of this hormone is unclear

Special cases in pituitary disease
What is pituitary apoplexy?
• This is caused by infarction of the pituitary gland, consequently resulting in failure of hormone production
• Can occur in patients with large pituitary tumours
• Any individual with known or suspected pituitary tumour complaining of sudden onset severe headache with or without cranial nerve palsies (III, IV and VI) should be suspected as having pituitary apoplexy
• Urgent MRI of the pituitary should be requested
• These patients should be given parenteral steroids
What is a craniopharyngioma?
• A tumour arising from the epithelial remnants of Rathke's pouch
• Can be present at any age and half the subjects are children
• Clinical presentation is similar to a non-functioning pituitary adenoma
• The presence of calcification in a pituitary tumour should raise the suspicion of a craniopharyngioma
• Treated surgically but recurrence rates are high
What is lymphocytic hypophysitis?
• A rare inflammatory condition of the pituitary, likely to be autoimmune in origin
• Results in pituitary hormonal failure and can cause a mass effect
• Spontaneous recovery may occur
• Usually treated with replacement of deficient hormone(s)

The thyroid

Anatomy
- The thyroid is composed of a midline isthmus just below the cricoid cartilage (Fig. 7), a right and a left lobe, extending from the isthmus laterally
- Thyroid cells are arranged in follicles and produce thyroid hormones, which are stored in the lumen of the follicle
- The thyroid also contains C cells, which produce calcitonin

Physiology
- Iodine is an essential component of thyroid hormones
- The thyroid gland traps iodine from the plasma, a process mediated by the sodium iodide symporter
- Iodine is then organified and iodothyronines (thyroid hormones) are formed, a process mediated by the enzyme thyroid peroxidase (TPO)
- Thyroid hormones are stored in thyroid follicles bound to thyroglobulin (TG)
- In response to demand, TG is internalized by thyroid follicular cells, and thyroid hormones are liberated into the blood stream
- Thyroid hormone secretion is constituted of 20% T3 and 80% T4
- T4 is converted in peripheral tissue to the active hormone T3, through the action of deiodinase enzymes
- Thyroid hormones are bound to plasma proteins (thyroxine binding globulin, albumin) and their levels can be influenced by plasma protein concentrations. Therefore, free thyroid hormone levels should be measured in cases of suspected thyroid hormone abnormalities
- Thyroid hormone production is regulated by the hypothalamus and pituitary gland as shown in Fig. 8.

Pathophysiology of the thyroid
Disorders of the thyroid gland include:
- Hormonal hypersecretion (hyperthyroidism): with or without thyroid gland enlargement (thyroid goitre)
- Hormonal hyposecretion (hypothyroidism): with or without thyroid goitre
- Thyroid nodules/goitre with normal thyroid hormone levels
- Thyroid cancers

An approach to a patient with suspected thyroid disease
A proper history is important particularly in relation to:
- Symptoms of hyper- or hypothyroidism (see below)
- In the case of thyroid nodules or goitre:
  - Recent change in size
  - Recent hoarse voice
  - Compressive symptoms (difficulty in breathing or swallowing)

Box 5 Examination of the thyroid

Assessment of thyroid status
- General
  - Is the patient fidgety or agitated?
  - Facial appearances
  - Is the patient's clothing appropriate? (Wearing a t-shirt in December suggests hyperthyroidism!)
- Hand tremor: best checked by placing a piece of paper on outstretched arms
- Sweaty or dry skin (check palms)
- Feel pulse (tachycardia, atrial fibrillation or bradycardia)
- Assess for lid lag
- Check for signs of proximal myopathy
- Tendon reflexes (ask the patient to kneel on a chair and check ankle reflexes)

Endocrinology and Diabetes: Clinical Cases Uncovered. By R. Ajjan.
Published 2009 by Blackwell Publishing, ISBN: 978-1-4051-5726-1

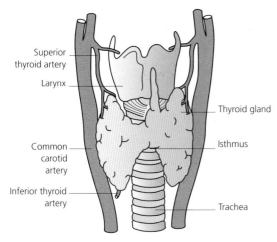

Figure 7 Anatomy of the thyroid gland. The isthmus of the gland thyroid is located just below the cricoid cartilage. The right and left lobes extend laterally and some individuals have a small conical lobe extending from the isthmus upwards called the pyramidal lobe.

Assessment of the thyroid gland

- Inspection
  - Observe for any neck swelling; ask the patient to swallow and observe for a neck mass that moves with swallowing
  - A midline structure moving by tongue protrusion suggests a thyroglossal cyst
- Palpation
  - Palpate the thyroid starting in the isthmus and moving out laterally and upwards. Use the pulp not the tip of your fingers
  - Feel the neck for lymphadenopathy
- Percussion: gives limited information about the possibility of retrosternal extension of a goitre
- Auscultation: bruit over the thyroid gland suggest a diagnosis of Graves' disease (due to increased gland vascularity)
- Check for Pemberton's sign: raising both arms above the head results in venous obstruction, which can be seen in large goitres with retrosternal extension
  Assessment for signs of extrathyroidal disease (in suspected Graves' disease)
- Graves' ophthalmopathy
  - Proptosis
  - Periorbital oedema
  - Conjunctival injection
  - Chemosis
  - Corneal ulceration
  - Inability to fully close the eyes
- Pretibial myxoedema
- Thyroid acropachy

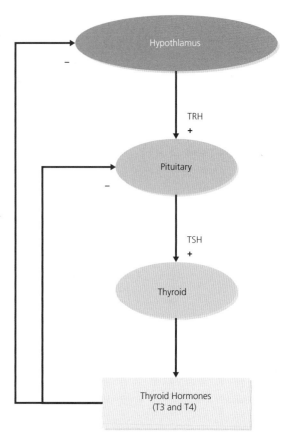

Figure 8 Regulation of thyroid hormone production. The hypothalamus produces thyrotropin releasing hormone (TRH), which stimulates the pituitary to secrete thyroid stimulating hormone (TSH), which in turn stimulates the thyroid gland to synthesize and release thyroid hormones. T3 and T4 have a negative feedback effect on TRH and TSH production.

Hyperthyroidism

Causes of hyperthyroidism are summarized in Table 6.

Graves' disease (GD)

- The commonest cause of hyperthyroidism (80% of cases)
- An autoimmune condition characterized by the presence of thyroid stimulating antibodies (TSAb), mimicking the action of TSH and resulting in hyperthyroidism
- Can be associated with extrathyroidal manifestations (summarized in Table 7, Fig. 9, colour plate section)

Clinical presentation

- Patient usually presents with classical symptoms hyperthyroidism (summarized in Table 8)

Table 6 Causes, aetiology and diagnosis of hyperthyroidism.

Cause of hyperthyroidism	Frequency and aetiology	Diagnosis
Graves' disease	80%, thyroid stimulating antibodies	Clinical examination
		Thyroid autoantibodies
		Thyroid uptake scan in uncertain cases
Toxic nodule or toxic multinodular goitre	15%, activating mutations in TSH receptor and Gsα protein	Clinical examination
		Thyroid uptake scan
Thyroiditis	2–4%, autoimmune, viral or drug-related (amiodarone)	Clinical examination
		Thyroid uptake scan
		ESR
TSH-secreting tumour	<1%	Raised TSH and thyroid hormones; pituitary imaging
Exogenous thyroid hormone administration	Variable, excess ingestion of thyroid hormones	Clinical assessment
Hyperemesis gravidarum	Rare, raised hCG (mimicking TSH action)	Clinical assessment
Choriocarcinoma		Absence of thyroid autoimmunity
		Known pregnancy
		Imaging of the pelvis
Struma ovarii	Rare, ectopic ovarian thyroid tissue	Clinical assessment
		Thyroid/pelvic uptake scan
		Imaging of the pelvis
Thyroid hormone resistance	Rare, pituitary resistance to thyroid hormones	Clinical assessment
		Family history

ESR, erythrocyte sedimentation rate; hCG, human chorionic gonadotrophins.

- Neck palpation reveals a smooth, uniform goitre in the majority of cases
- Around half the patients will have extrathyroidal manifestations of the disease (summarized in Table 7 and shown in Fig. 9 and Fig. 40)

Investigations
- Confirm the presence of hyperthyroidism:
  - Suppressed TSH
  - Raised thyroid hormones (T4 and/or T3)
  - Detection of thyroid stimulating antibodies: not essential for making the diagnosis and usually reserved for atypical cases. These are positive in 95–99% of GD cases depending on the type of assay used
- In uncertain cases (no or asymmetrical goitre, negative antibodies):
  - Thyroid uptake scan: in Graves' disease this shows uniform uptake of technetium or iodine (Fig. 10)

Treatment
GD can be treated with antithyroid drugs, radioactive iodine and surgery. Symptomatic treatment is also possible in patients with severe symptoms; β-adrenergic blocking agents (propranolol) can be used but these are only required in a minority.

Antithyroid drugs (thionamides)
- Include propylthiouracil, carbimazole and its active metabolite methimazole
- These agents interfere with the action of thyroid peroxidase, thereby inhibiting thyroid hormone production

Table 7 Extrathyroidal manifestations of Graves' disease. Extrathyroidal disease, usually Graves' ophthalmopathy (GO) can be seen even in individuals with normal thyroid function.

Extrathyroidal manifestations of Graves' disease	Clinical findings
Graves' ophthalmopathy	Clinically evident in 50% of Graves' disease patients but can be seen in 90% using imaging techniques
	Characterized by swelling of the extraorbital muscles and proliferation of adipose and connective tissue in the orbit
	The above results in proptosis of the eyes and in severe cases exposure keratitis. Also, it may result in ophthalmoplegia and optic neuropathy
Graves' dermopathy	Rare, usually affects the shins (hence pretibial myxoedema)
	Skin looks discoloured, indurated and can be itchy
	Graves' dermopathy is almost always associated with GO
Graves' acropachy	Very rare, usually associated with GO and Graves' dermopathy
	Characterized by clubbing and subperiosteal new bone formation

Table 8 Symptoms and signs of Graves' disease. Hyperthyroidism due to other causes presents with similar symptoms and signs except for the absence of GO, PTM and acropachy.

Symptoms	Frequency
Nervousness, heat intolerance and perspiration, palpitations, fatigue	85–95%
Increased frequency of stools, weight loss with increased appetite	75–85%
Symptoms of Graves' ophthalmopathy	50%
Insomnia, polyuria and menstrual irregularities	20–30%

Signs	Frequency
Hyperkinetic behaviour, tachycardia or atrial fibrillation	90–95%
Goitre, warm and moist skin, hand tremor	90%
Signs of Graves' ophthalmopathy	50%
Pretibial myxoedema	5%
Onycholysis, acropachy	<5%

Rare presentations

Thyroid storm: an extreme form of thyrotoxicosis presenting with fever, cardiovascular collapse, confusion, psychosis, severe weakness and even coma. This is a life-threatening emergency that requires urgent medical treatment (see text).

Apathetic hyperthyroidism: the adrenergic hyperactivity manifestations are absent and this presentation can be confused with depression (usually occurs in the elderly).

- Antithyroid drugs can be given as
  - Titration regime (usually for 18 months): enough antithyroid drug is given to keep the thyroid hormones in the normal range
  - Block and replace regime (usually for 6 months): a large dose of antithyroid drug is given to fully block thyroid hormone production and thyroxine replacement therapy is added to ensure adequate plasma thyroid hormone levels
  - After 6–18 months, treatment is stopped and disease remission is achieved in less than 50%

Radioactive iodine (RAI)
- Safe and effective treatment (up to 90% respond after one dose)
- Used as second line in Europe but frequently as first line in America

> **Box 6 Side effects of antithyroid drugs**
>
> - Agranulocytosis: the most serious complication and all patients are advised to immediately report to their physician in case they develop a temperature, sore throat or mouth ulcers. Agranulocytosis with either propylthiouracil or carbimazole represents a contraindication to the use of these agents
> - Minor side effects such as rash, musculoskeletal pain, deranged liver function. If these occur, it is possible to switch between antithyroid drugs

- RAI treatment destroys the thyroid gland and can take up to 6 months to have full effect

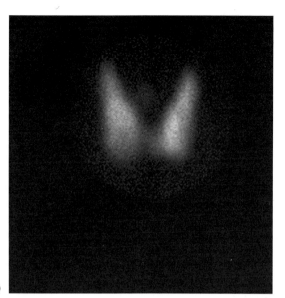

(a)

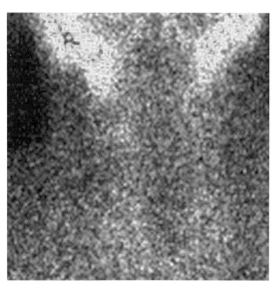

(b)

Figure 10 Technetium scan in an individual with Graves' disease, demonstrating uniform uptake and thyroiditis showing lack of uptake. Courtesy of Dr R. Bury, the Radionuclide Department, University of Leeds.

• Induces long-term hypothyroidism (patients need to be warned that they will potentially need lifelong treatment with thyroxine)
• Contraindications include:
  ◦ Absolute: pregnancy
  ◦ Relative: active eye disease (eye disease may worsen after RAI)

Surgery
This is reserved for those with:
• Large goitre
• Personal preference
• Severe hyperthyroidism and intolerance to antithyroid drugs

Toxic solitary nodule (TN) and toxic multinodular goitre (TMNG)

Around 15% of hyperthyroid patients have a TN or TMNG.

Clinical presentation
• Symptoms and signs of hyperthyroidism
• Neck palpation reveals an irregular goitre or a thyroid nodule
• There are no extrathyroidal signs

Investigations
• Confirm the presence of biochemical hyperthyroidism
• Thyroid uptake scan shows one or more thyroid nodules with increased uptake, which are often referred to as "hot" nodules
• Hyperthyroidism due to toxic nodule(s) must be differentiated from GD and a cold nodule (an uptake scan can be used), due to the relatively high prevalence of malignancy in GD-associated cold nodules
• A thyroid uptake scan for a toxic nodule is shown in (Fig. 11)

Treatment
• Toxic solitary nodule or toxic multinodular goitre can be treated with antithyroid drugs but the disease relapses once medical treatment is stopped
• The best treatment option is radioactive iodine, which often restores euthyroidism
• Surgery is also an option but is reserved for a minority of patients, usually those with large disfiguring goitres
• Fine needle aspiration (FNA) is only required in selected cases (malignancy in toxic nodules is rare) and this is discussed below

Thyroiditis
• A relatively rare cause of hyperthyroidism
• May be autoimmune in nature, follow a viral disease or can be drug-related

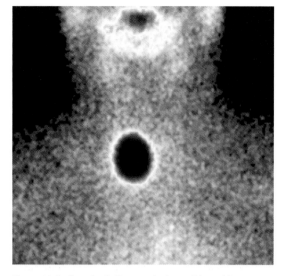

Figure 11 Radioactive iodine uptake in a subject with hyperthyroidism shows a toxic nodule with suppression of uptake activity in the rest of the gland. Courtesy of Dr. R. Bury the Radionuclide Department, University of Leeds.

Table 9 Symptoms and signs of hypothyroidism.

Symptoms	Frequency
Weakness/lethargy, dry skin	95%
Sensation of cold and decreased sweating, oedema of the face	80%
Impaired memory, constipation, hair loss and weight gain	65%
Deafness and non-specific chest pain	30%

Signs	Frequency
Thick tongue, facial oedema, dry and cold skin	80%
Slow relaxing reflexes	75%
Bradycardia, skin pallor, coarse hair, depression	60%

Clinical presentation

• Symptoms and signs of thyrotoxicosis as discussed above

• Commonly secondary to a viral infection; therefore, thyrotoxic symptoms following a flu-like illness should raise the suspicion of thyroiditis

• Individuals may experience pain and tenderness in the region of the thyroid gland, a condition called De Quervain thyroiditis

• Diagnosis is made by demonstrating biochemical thyrotoxicosis, associated with lack of uptake on thyroid scan (Fig. 10)

• Postpartum thyroiditis
  ○ Occurs in 5–10% of women within 1 year of delivery
  ○ Characterized by a hyperthyroid phase within 4–6 months of delivery followed by a hypothyroid phase with subsequent restoration of normal thyroid function
  ○ Permanent hypothyroidism eventually develops in around one-third of patients

Treatment

• The disease is self-limiting and treatment is not usually required

• For neck pain and tenderness, non-steroidal anti-inflammatory agents can be used, whereas steroids are reserved for severe cases

• Thyrotoxic phase is usually followed by a hypothyroid phase, which may require a short course of thyroid hormone replacement until the thyroid follicular cells are fully recovered

Hyperthyroidism secondary to TSH-secreting tumours (TSH-oma)

• This is a rare cause of hyperthyroidism

• It should be suspected in individuals with raised thyroid hormones and detectable TSH levels

• TSH-oma is discussed in the pituitary section

Hypothyroidism

A common disease, mainly affecting the female population. Causes include:

• Autoimmune hypothyroidism: by far the commonest cause
  ○ Atrophic (no goitre palpable)
  ○ Goitrous (Hashimoto's thyroiditis)

• Postpartum thyroiditis

• Post-radiation

• Iodine deficiency

• Drugs (amiodarone, lithium)

• Congenital developmental and biosynthetic defects

• Secondary (due to pituitary or hypothalamic defects)

Clinical presentation

This can be very variable and the commonest symptoms and signs are summarized in Table 9.

Investigations

- Biochemical testing shows low plasma thyroid hormone levels with raised TSH
- Some individuals may have high TSH with normal thyroid hormone levels, a condition known as subclinical hypothyroidism which is discussed below
- Thyroid antibodies (TPO antibodies) are usually detected in individuals with autoimmune hypothyroidism
- Any subject with low plasma thyroid hormone levels with low or normal TSH should be suspected of having secondary hypothyroidism (i.e. pituitary failure) and urgent investigations/endocrine referral should be made

Treatment

- This is relatively simple and consists of replacing thyroid hormone
- L-thyroxine (T4) is usually given, which is converted in the periphery to the active hormone T3
- Combination therapy with T3 and T4 is very rarely used and only in selected patients who remain symptomatic on T4 replacement alone
- The appropriate dose of thyroxine should titrated to suppress TSH below 2 mIU/L but full suppression should be avoided (usual replacement dose is around 1.4 mcg/kg)

Special cases of abnormal thyroid function
Subclinical hypothyroidism (SHypo)

- Raised TSH levels in the presence of normal thyroid hormones is defined as SHypo
- SHypo is usually due to early autoimmune hypothyroidism
- The term SHypo suggests the absence of symptoms but this is somewhat misleading as a large proportion of these patients are symptomatic
- Thyroid function should be repeated within 3 months and if TSH remains elevated (or it is increasing), then treatment is advised, particularly in patients with positive TPO antibodies
- Some studies suggest an association between subclinical hypothyroidism and atherosclerotic disease
- The aim of treatment is to normalize TSH

Subclinical hyperthyroidism (SHyper)

- Suppressed TSH with normal thyroid hormone levels (both T4 and T3) is defined as SHyper

- It may be due to:
  - Graves' disease
  - Toxic multinodular goitre
- Usually occurs in older individuals who may display mild symptoms of hyperthyroidism but may be asymptomatic
- Subjects with SHyper are at increased risk of:
  - Atrial fibrillation
  - Osteoporosis
- Radioactive iodine is usually the best treatment option for these individuals

Amiodarone-induced thyroid dysfunction

This can be a difficult condition to manage even for an experienced endocrinologist. Amiodarone can result in both hypo- and hyperthyroidism through:

- High iodine content of the drug (40% of its weight)
- Direct toxic effect of amiodarone on thyroid follicular cells

Amiodarone-induced hypothyroidism

- Occurs in up to 15% of patients on the drug
- This can be simply managed by giving thyroid hormone replacement similarly to individual with primary hypothyroidism
- Discontinuation of amiodarone (which is not always possible) can result in restoration of normal thyroid function

Amiodarone-induced hyperthyroidism (AIT)

This occurs in less than 5% of patients on amiodarone treatment, and can be divided into:

- AIT type I
  - Similar to autoimmune hyperthyroidism
  - Can be managed with antithyroid drugs
  - RAI is usually ineffective (need to stop amiodarone for a year before considering RAI)
  - Thyroidectomy should be considered for difficult cases
- AIT type II
  - This is due to thyroiditis and thyroid destruction
  - Usually managed with high doses of steroids
- Mixed type I and type II AIT can occur and is best managed by a combination of antithyroid drugs and steroids
- Amiodarone withdrawal is advisable in subjects with AIT but this is not always possible

Any patient planned for amiodarone treatment should have:

Table 10 Important characteristics of type I and type II AIT.

	Type I AIT	Type II AIT
Goitre	Frequent	Rare
Thyroid antibodies	Positive	Negative
Plasma CRP	Normal	High
Plasma IL-6	Normal	High
Vascularity (Doppler studies)	Increased	Reduced

CRP, C-reactive protein.

• Thyroid function and thyroid antibody screen done prior to starting treatment
• Thyroid function tested every 6 months whilst on this therapy and for 12 months after discontinuing the drug
   Table 10 summarizes the important characteristics of type I and type II AIT.

Thyroid storm

A rare, severe and life-threatening case of hyperthyroidism characterized by:
• Reduced conscious level
• Hyperthermia
• Multisystem decompensation (cardiac failure, renal failure, etc.)
   Treatment consists of:
• High-dose antithyroid drugs
• Potassium iodine
• β-blockers
• Steroids

Myoedema coma

A rare, severe and life-threatening case of hypothyroidism.
• Often precipitated by infection
• Characterized by:
   ○ Reduced conscious levels
   ○ Hypothermia
   ○ Respiratory depression and associated CO_2 retention
• Treatment consists of:
   ○ T3 and T4
   ○ Antibiotic cover after appropriate cultures
   ○ Steroid cover (associated adrenal dysfunction is common)

Hypo- and hyperthyroidism during pregnancy

• Hypothyroidism in pregnancy

   ○ The dose of thyroxine replacement is usually increased in pregnancy by up to 50%
   ○ Thyroid hormone levels should be kept at the upper end of normal (without TSH suppression) in women with hypothyroidism receiving thyroxine replacement during pregnancy
• Graves' disease in pregnancy
   ○ Block and replace is contraindicated (antithyroid drugs cross the placenta whereas thyroxine does not, potentially resulting in fetal hypothyroidism)
• Propylthiouracil is probably safer to use than carbimazole due to reported congenital abnormalities with the latter
• The lowest dose of antithyroid drugs should be used to keep thyroid hormones at the upper end of normal range

Thyroid nodular disease in euthyroid subjects (thyroid nodules and multinodular goitre)

• Very common, clinically evident in around 10% of the UK population
• A thyroid goitre can be physiological:
   ○ Puberty
   ○ Pregnancy
• Non-physiological causes of thyroid goitre include:
   ○ Thyroid autoimmunity
   ○ Iodine deficiency (endemic goitre)
   ○ Drugs (lithium)
   ○ Other (unknown)
• A thyroid nodule can be:
   ○ Solid: composed of thyroid tissue
   ○ Cystic: usually filled with brown fluid
   ○ Mixed: solid/cystic
• Thyroid nodules/goitres are more common in women
• Only a minority of thyroid nodules are malignant (<5%)
• Thyroid nodules are more likely to be malignant in:
   ○ Young (<20 years) or older (>60 years) subjects
   ○ Rapidly growing nodule
   ○ Compressive symptoms: hoarse voice, dysphagia, breathing difficulties
   ○ Family history of endocrine malignancy
   ○ Cold nodule in an individual with Graves' disease
   ○ History of familial polyposis coli (papillary carcinoma), Hirshprung's disease (medullary thyroid cancer) or Hashimoto's thyroiditis (thyroid lymphoma)

Table 11 Classification of thyroid cancers.

Characteristics	Papillary	Follicular	Anaplastic	Medullary*	Lymphoma
Cell type	Thyroid cells	Thyroid cells	Thyroid cells	C cells	Lymphocytes
Age at presentation	30–50	40–50	>60	Any age	>40
Frequency	75%	15%	<5%	<5%	<5%
Prognosis	Good	Good	Very poor	Variable	Variable
Treatment	Surgery and RAI ablation	Surgery and RAI ablation	Surgery Chemotherapy External radiation	Surgery	Chemotherapy radiation

*May be part of MEN II or familial medullary carcinoma and is associated with raised serum calcitonin levels.

PART 1: BASICS

Clinical presentation

Patient presents with a history of lump in the neck, which is:

- Observed by the patient
- Observed by a family member/friend
- Detected during investigations for other pathologies (ultrasound or CT neck)

Alarming features include:

- Predisposition to thyroid malignancy as above
- Rapidly growing goitre or nodule
- Compressive symptoms or hoarse voice
- Very hard nodule
- Fixation of skin above the nodule
- Presence of neck lymphadenopathy

Investigations of thyroid nodules/multinodular goitre

- Fine needle aspiration (FNA) of the solitary nodule or dominant nodule in a multinodular. A simple test, usually done in a clinic
  - Benign cytology: follow-up with repeat FNA in 6 months is required
  - Inconclusive: repeat FNA (if repeat is undetermined then refer to surgery)
  - Features of malignancy: surgery
- CT scan in large goitres and in the presence of compressive symptoms
- Pulmonary function tests to establish the presence of respiratory compromise

Treatment

- Clinically and/or cytologically suspicious nodules should be treated with surgery, followed by radioactive iodine ablation (high doses of radioactive iodine) if histology confirms malignancy (up to 10% of FNA gives false-positive results)
- Nodules with benign cytology can be followed up medically with regular examination and repeat FNA as necessary

Thyroid cancers

- Thyroid cancers are rare and mortality is low as most carry a good prognosis
- Occur more commonly in women but a thyroid nodule in man is more likely to be malignant
- Risk factors and indicators of malignancy in thyroid nodules are discussed above
- Classification of thyroid cancers is summarized in Table 11

Clinical presentation

- A thyroid nodule or goitre: a rapidly growing thyroid nodule should raise the suspicion of malignancy
- Post-mortem examination has shown that thyroid cancers are not uncommon and individuals die with, rather than from, the disease
- Risk factors for thyroid cancers should be elicited in the history
- Hard nodules and cervical lymphadenopathy should raise the suspicion of malignancy

Investigations

- FNA as above
- Ensure that patient is not thyrotoxic before performing FNA

Treatment

Patients with cytologically proven papillary or follicular thyroid malignancy should undergo:

- Total thyroidectomy
- Radioactive iodine ablation
- This should be followed by treatment with TSH-suppressive doses of thyroxine (i.e. supraphysiological doses of throxine are given to keep TSH suppressed)

Patients with medullary carcinoma should undergo:

- Total thyroidectomy and lymph node dissection
- Suppressive therapy with thyroxine is not needed (C cells are not controlled by TSH)
- Appropriate testing should be arranged to rule out MEN II (see neuroendocrine section)

Anaplastic carcinoma

- Prognosis is very poor and surgery is rarely successful
- Palliative radiotherapy can be arranged, whereas chemotherapy is generally ineffective

Lymphoma

- Usually treated with radio- and chemotherapy

Patients with strong clinical suspicion of malignancy but negative FNA should still be considered for surgery as FNA can give false-negative results in a minority of cases (5–10%).

Patients with previous thyroid cancer should be monitored for life

- Regular examination
- Thyroglobulin plasma levels: detectable thyroglobulin plasma levels after surgery and radioactive ablation therapy indicate the presence of residual thyroid tissue and, hence, recurrence of the disease

Bone and calcium metabolism

Parathyroid hormone (PTH), secreted by the parathyroid glands, is the main hormone responsible for calcium haemostasis. There are five organs involved in calcium metabolism:
- Parathyroid gland, through the secretion of PTH, which increases plasma calcium levels
- Gastrointestinal tract (absorption of calcium)
- Renal tract (excretion of calcium)
- Bone (storage of calcium)
- Thyroid gland, through the secretion of calcitonin by C cells
  ○ Calcitonin has a weak calcium-lowering effect
  ○ Plasma calcitonin levels are only used for the diagnosis of medullary thyroid cancer and have no role in investigations of disorders of calcium metabolism

Anatomy
Usually, there are four parathyroid glands located at the back of the thyroid gland (see Fig. 12). Rarely, ectopic parathyroid tissue can be identified in the thoracic cavity, which is due to abnormal parathyroid gland migration during embryogenesis.

Physiology
Bones are in constant turnover, through the action of:
- Osteoclasts: these cells are responsible for bone resorption
- Osteoblasts: these are responsible for bone formation
  Calcium is important for:
- Bone health
- Neuromuscular conduction
  Plasma calcium levels, which should always be corrected for plasma albumin, are kept in check by a number of mechanisms/organs:
- Parathyroid gland: PTH results in calcium liberation

from bone, increased intestinal absorption and reduced urinary excretion, and, hence, increases plasma calcium levels (low blood calcium levels result in increased secretion of PTH, whereas high levels lead to suppression of PTH release)
- Gastrointestinal tract: Vitamin D plays an important role in controlling absorption of calcium in the gut
  ○ Vitamin D undergoes 25-hydroxylation and 1-hydroxylation in the liver and kidneys, respectively, to form active vitamin D [1,25-$(OH)_2$D]
  ○ Vitamin D enhances intestinal calcium absorption
- Kidneys: calcium is reabsorbed by the kidneys, a process regulated by PTH
- PTH results in increased calcium and decreased phosphate reabsorption (i.e. phosphate loss) by the kidneys. Therefore, in primary hyperparathyroidism, hypercalcaemia is often associated with hypophosphataemia

Pathophysiology
- Hypocalcaemia and hypercalcaemia are relatively common clinical conditions and are discussed below
- Osteoporosis is characterized by an increase in osteoclast over osteoblast activity, resulting in reduction in bone mass (quantitative change), consequently predisposing to fractures
- Osteomalacia is characterized by insufficient calcium in bone tissue with normal bone mass (qualitative change)
- In Paget's disease, the activity of osteoblasts and osteoclasts is disorganized resulting in both bone resorption and new bone formation in an uncoordinated manner
  This chapter will discuss a number of different clinical entities including:
- Hypocalcaemia
- Hypercalcaemia
- Osteomalacia and rickets
- Osteoporosis
- Paget's disease
- Inherited bone abnormalities

Endocrinology and Diabetes: Clinical Cases Uncovered. By R. Ajjan.
Published 2009 by Blackwell Publishing, ISBN: 978-1-4051-5726-1

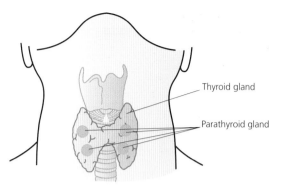

Figure 12 The four parathyroid glands are located on the posterior aspect of the thyroid gland.

Thyroid gland

Parathyroid gland

Hypocalcaemia

This is not an uncommon condition and causes include:
- Vitamin D deficiency: probably the commonest cause, secondary to:
  ○ Poor sunlight exposure (commonly seen in Asian women who cover their bodies with clothes)
  ○ Malabsorption (coeliac disease is a common cause)
  ○ Poor diet (frequently seen in the elderly)
  ○ Kidney disease (failure of 1-hydroxylation of vitamin D)
- Hypoparathyroidism
  ○ Congenital
  ○ Destruction of the glands by radiation, surgery or autoimmunity
- Hypomagnesaemia (inhibits PTH secretion), which may be due to:
  ○ Gastrointestinal loss
  ○ Renal loss
  ○ Drugs (diuretics, cyclosporine, alcohol)
- Drugs
  ○ Calcitonin
- Increased calcium uptake by bone
  ○ Hungry bone syndrome (following thyroid or para-thyroid surgery)
  ○ Osteoblastic bony metastasis (prostate cancer)
- Complexing of calcium from the circulation
  ○ Acute pancreatitis (calcium soap formation due to fat autodigestion)
  ○ Multiple blood transfusions (complex of calcium with citrate)
- Functional: inability of PTH to exert its effect (PTH resistance), also known as pseudohypoparathyroidism

Clinical presentation

This can be variable from one person to another and is related to the degree of hypocalcaemia. Symptoms include:
- Tingling and numbness (often described by the patient as pins and needles sensation) in the fingers, toes and lips
- Cramps
- In severe cases, stridor (due to spasm of laryngeal muscles) and/or seizures

Low calcium results in neuromuscular irritability and, therefore, the following signs can be found:
- Chvostek's sign: tapping on the facial nerve in front of the ear results in twitching of the corner of the mouth
- Trousseau's sign: inflation of the sphygmomanometer above the arterial pressure results in carpopedal spasm

Investigations

- Plasma calcium: diagnosis is confirmed by demonstrating low plasma calcium (make sure corrected calcium levels are assessed)
- Establish the cause:
  ○ Check PTH levels: low PTH levels in the presence of hypocalcaemia indicate parathyroid failure
  ○ Vitamin D levels: patients with low vitamin D levels should be investigated for the possibility of coeliac disease
  ○ Renal function
  ○ Magnesium levels

Treatment

- Acute symptomatic hypocalcaemia (tetany, seizures) is a medical emergency and should be treated with i.v. calcium
  ○ 20 mL of 10% calcium diluted in 100–200 saline should be infused over 10–20 min
  ○ Further calcium infusion may be needed (24 h slow calcium infusion is frequently used)
  ○ Regular monitoring of calcium levels should be organized (every 4–8 h)
  ○ Care should be taken against extravasation of calcium into interstitial tissue, which may cause necrosis (a large vein should be used for i.v. calcium administration)
  ○ Intravenous treatment should be followed by oral calcium administration and correction of the precipitating cause

- Acute hypocalcaemia with mild symptoms
  - Oral therapy with calcium and vitamin D is usually given
  - Correction of the underlying cause
  - Patient should be carefully monitored
- Chronic hypocalcaemia
  - Treatment should be directed at correcting the underlying cause

Hypercalcaemia

Hypercalcaemia is commonly seen on the general medical wards. Causes include:

- Increased secretion of PTH
  - Primary hyperparathyroidism
  - Tertiary hyperparathyroidism
- Malignancy
  - Secretion of PTH-related peptide
  - Bony invasion in metastatic disease
- Familial, e.g. familial hypocalciuric hypercalcaemia (secondary to low urinary calcium excretion)
  - Autosomal dominant disease due to mutation in the calcium-sensing receptor
  - PTH levels are usually in the normal range
  - It must be differentiated from primary hyperparathyroidism, otherwise the patient may undergo unnecessary surgery
  - Patient usually asymptomatic and diagnosis is made by demonstrating reduced urinary calcium excretion with high plasma calcium
- Medications
  - Thiazide diuretics
  - Vitamin D intoxication
  - Vitamin A intoxication
- Granulomatous disease
  - Sarcoidosis
- Endocrine causes (rare)
  - Hyperthyroidism
  - Addison's disease
  - Acromegaly

Clinical presentation

Symptoms are usually insidious and include:

- Osmotic symptoms
  - Polyuria
  - Polydipsia
  - Dehydration
- Gastrointestinal
  - Anorexia and vomiting
  - Abdominal pain
  - Constipation
- Central nervous system
  - Confusion
  - Depression

Investigations

- Plasma calcium levels: these are elevated (make sure corrected calcium levels are used)
- PTH
  - Raised: hyperparathyroidism
  - Suppressed: non-parathyroid cause
  - Normal: early hyperparathyroidism (usually calcium levels are only mildly elevated) or familial hypocalciuric hypercalcaemia (FHH)
- Establish the cause
  - History and full examination: this is important as it may give clues to the presence of a malignant disorder
  - In those with elevated PTH, the most likely diagnosis is a parathyroid adenoma and localization of this can be done with: CT scan of the neck and chest, ultrasound of the neck and ^{99m}Tc-cestamibi scan, which relies on concentration of the radioactive material in the parathyroid tissue
  - Renal function: chronic renal failure may result in tertiary hyperparathyroidism
  - Chest X-ray: particularly in those with respiratory symptoms (exclude a malignant lung condition)
  - Myeloma screen: hypercalcaemia can be one of the early manifestations of multiple myeloma
  - Vitamin D levels: to rule out vitamin D intoxication
  - 24-h urinary calcium: low urinary calcium excretion in FHH (important to make this diagnosis as no treatment is usually required)
  - In case of suspicion, rule out endocrine causes of hypercalcaemia: hyperthyroidism (TFTs), adrenal failure (synacthen test) and acromegaly (glucose tolerance test, if history is suggestive)
- Determine end organ damage
  - Ultrasound of the renal tract
  - Skeletal radiographs
  - Check bone mineral density

Treatment

For severe symptomatic hypercalcaemia:

- Rehydrate patient with i.v. fluid

- Intravenous bisphosphonates (pamidronate is frequently used): these agents should only be given after adequate hydration
- Treat the cause of hypercalcaemia
- In resistant cases calcitonin can be used

For moderate hypercalcaemia:
- Ensure adequate patient hydration
- Treat the underlying cause:
  ○ Surgery for hyperparathyroidism: in mild cases, this is not always necessary and patient can be simply followed up with regular calcium checks and monitoring for end organ damage
- Hypercalcaemia of malignancy may partly respond to systemic steroids, which can be given until specific cancer treatment is introduced

Osteomalacia and rickets

Osteomalacia and rickets are due to inadequate mineralization of bone. The former occurs in mature bone, whereas the latter occurs in growing bone. Causes of osteomalacia and rickets include:

- Associated with low phosphate
  ○ Vitamin D deficiency (the commonest cause): low phosphate is due to increased PTH secretion
  ○ Vitamin D-dependent rickets: due to deficient vitamin D receptor or inadequate conversion of vitamin D to the active form (rare)
  ○ Excessive loss of urinary phosphate (rare): oncogenic osteomalacia (seen in malignant disease), X-linked hypophosphataemia, renal tubular acidosis and drugs (diuretics)
  ○ Decreased phosphate availability: starvation, malnutrition (alcoholism in the UK is one cause) and malabsorption
- Associated with high phosphate
  ○ Renal failure

The vast majority of patients will have osteomalacia/rickets due to vitamin D deficiency with or without renal disease, this is what you need to remember.

Clinical presentation

Symptoms and signs of osteomalacia/rickets are summarized in Table 12.

Investigations
- Calcium: low or low-normal
- Phosphate: usually low, except for osteomalacia due to renal failure

Table 12 Symptoms and signs of osteomalacia and rickets.

Osteomalacia	Rickets
Bone pain	Growth retardation
Fractures	Bone pain and fractures
Proximal myopathy	Skeletal deformities:
	Bowing of tibia
	Rickety rosary
	Widening of wrists

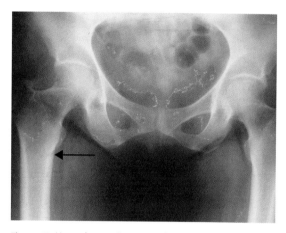

Figure 13 X-ray changes in osteomalacia. A partial fracture in the femur, known as a Looser zone or pseudofracture, can be seen in subjects with osteomalacia.

- PTH: usually elevated (except for some rare causes of osteomalacia)
- Vitamin D levels
- Bone X-ray
  ○ Pseudofractures or Looser zones: these are pathognomic of osteomalacia (see Fig. 13)
  ○ Widening of growth plates and bone deformity: seen in rickets

Table 13 summarizes the biochemical findings in common causes of osteomalacia/rickets.

Treatment
- Vitamin D replacement
  ○ Calciferol can be given orally often with calcium supplementation

Table 13 Biochemical findings in osteomalacia/rickets caused by vitamin D deficiency and renal failure. It is important to remember that longstanding renal failure can be associated with hypercalcaemia (rather than hypocalcaemia) due to tertiary hyperparathyroidism.

	Calcium	Phosphate	Alkaline phosphatase	25-OH-Vit D	PTH
Vit D deficiency (dietary, malabsorption)	↓	↓	↑	↓	↑
Renal failure	↓	↑	↑	N	↑

○ In renal failure 1-OH vitamin D (1-α-calciferol) should be given as the kidneys are unable to convert 25-OH vitamin D to the active 1, 25-OH vitamin D
• Treat the underlying cause

Osteoporosis
• This is a very common condition, which is due to a reduction in bone mass

---

Box 7 Loss of bone mass and osteoporosis

• From the age of 40, there is a gradual loss in bone mass (around 0.5% annually)
• Due to the protective effects of sex hormones, osteoporosis is common in women after the menopause and is called postmenopausal osteoporosis
• In women, bone mass loss after the menopause is accelerated, which explains the higher rate of osteoporotic fractures in older women compared with men

---

Causes include:
• Gonadal failure
  ○ Women: premature menopause (physiological menopause in the older age group) and any cause of amenorrhoea
  ○ Men: Kleinfelter's syndrome and acquired hypogonadism
• Drugs (long-term use)
  ○ Steroids
  ○ Heparin
  ○ Anticonvulsants
• Gastrointestinal and nutritional
  ○ Malabsorption due to any cause (for example coeliac disease)
  ○ Malnutrition (excessive alcohol, anorexia nervosa)
• Endocrine disease
  ○ Hyperparathyroidism
  ○ Cushing's syndrome

○ Hyperthyroidism
○ Growth hormone deficiency
• Inflammatory conditions
  ○ Rheumatoid arthritis
• Neoplastic disease
  ○ Multiple myeloma

Clinical presentation
The disease is usually silent until the occurrence of fractures (it does not cause skeletal pain).
• Low trauma fractures are a common presentation
• Vertebral fractures are also common resulting in:
  ○ Back pain (usually sudden onset and well localized)
  ○ Loss of height (this explains why older individuals shrink in size!)
  ○ Kyphosis
  ○ Spinal cord compression in severe cases

Investigations
Measure bone mineral density (BMD) using dual energy X-ray absorptiometry (known as DEXA scan):
Establish the cause

Box 8 Bone mineral density (BMD)

• BMD > −1: normal
• BMD < −1 but > −2.5: osteopenia
• BMD < −2.5: osteoporosis

• Full blood count (FBC), ESR (rule out inflammatory condition)
• Calcium levels
• Renal function
• Thyroid function
• Testosterone levels in men
• Oestradiol and FSH/LH levels in women with early menopause
• X-rays to rule out fractures. Back X-rays (see Fig. 14) are requested to rule out vertebral crush fractures in

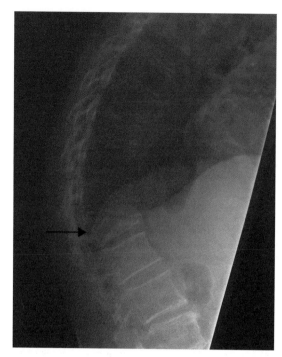

Figure 14 The x-ray shows a crush fracture of the vertebral body (can be seen as shorter vertebral body with increased bone density). In the presence of a crush fracture, DEXA scan may be inaccurate in measuring vertebral bone density.

those with: significant loss of height and/or sudden-onset back pain.
• More tests may be required to exclude specific conditions

Treatment
• Hormone replacement therapy (HRT)
  ○ Postmenopausal women
  ○ Women with gonadal failure
• Testosterone replacement
  ○ Men with gonadal failure
• Calcium and vitamin D
• Bisphosphonates: remain the mainstay of osteoporosis treatment usually in combination with calcium and vitamin D
• Strontium can be effective but makes BMD measurements unreliable (the drug is incorporated into the bone structure)
• Calcitonin can be effective in those with vertebral crush fractures as it partially relieves the pain
• Treatment is monitored
  ○ Clinically: no further fractures/loss of height
  ○ Repeat BMD 1–2 years after starting the treatment

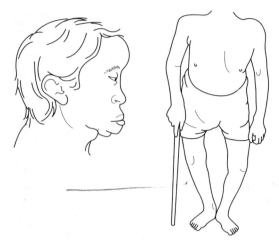

Figure 15 Typical "frontal bossing" and bowing of the bones.

Paget's disease
The main abnormality in Paget's disease is overactivity of the osteoblasts resulting in bone resorption. This in turn stimulates osteoblast function resulting in the formation of new bone. Bone resorption and formation is disorganized, consequently leading to bony deformities.

Clinical presentation
Paget's disease mainly affects the skull, vertebrae, pelvis, femur and tibia. Therefore, the patient presents with:
• Bone deformities (skull abnormalities, bowing of tibia) (see Fig. 15)
• Bone pain
• Fractures
• Complications
  ○ Nerve compression (may result in deafness)
  ○ Spinal cord compression (may result in paralysis)
  ○ Sarcomatous transformation (osteogenic sarcoma): fortunately, a rare event
  It should be noted that the vast majority of patients (up to 90%) are asymptomatic and the disease is diagnosed during routine laboratory investigations (raised alkaline phosphatase).

Investigations
• Alkaline phosphatase: usually elevated and can reach very high levels
• Bone X-ray:
  ○ Lytic (bone resorption) lesions
  ○ Sclerotic (new bone formation) lesions (Fig. 16)
• Bone isotope scan: helpful to fully assess the extent of bony involvement (Fig. 17)

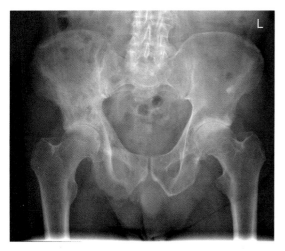

Figure 16 Typical lytic and sclerotic lesions in Paget's disease of the pelvis.

Treatment
- High dose oral bisphosphonate is the mainstay of treatment
- Indications for treatment include:
  - Bone pain
  - Neurological complications
  - Fractures
  - Hypercalcaemia (which is a rare complication of Paget's disease)
- Monitoring therapy
  - Clinical improvement
  - Alkaline phosphatase levels: these usually fall with successful treatment

Osteogenesis imperfecta
- A familial disease that can be inherited as autosomal dominant (AD) or autosomal recessive (AR)
- Several mutations are recognized leading to different clinical presentations

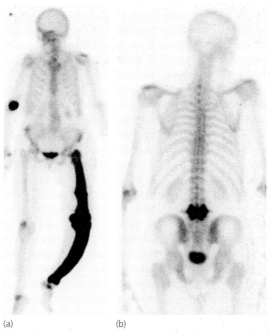

(a)   (b)

Figure 17 An isotope bone scan showing an increased uptake in the left femur and tibia, and right elbow and (b) vertebral body. Courtesy of Dr R. Bury, Radionuclide Department, University of Leeds.

- Main abnormality is in bone architecture, resulting in:
  - Severe osteoporosis and easy fractures: these individuals usually develop multiple fractures during their lifetime
  - Associated abnormalities include: blue sclera, abnormalities in teeth and hearing loss

Treatment
- Bisphosphonates can partly help by:
  - Increasing bone mass
  - Reducing the incidence of fractures

The adrenal glands

Anatomy
- The adrenal glands are situated above the kidneys (Fig. 18)
- The aorta and renal arteries provide the arterial blood supply to the adrenal glands, whereas venous drainage usually occurs into the inferior vena cava on the right and left renal vein on the left
- The adrenal glands are composed of:
  - Adrenal cortex, which represents 90% of the gland and produces corticosteroids (cortisol), mineralocorticoid (aldosterone) and androgens [dehydroepiandrosterone (DHEA) and androstenedione]
  - Adrenal medulla, which represents 10% of the adrenal gland and produces catecholamines (adrenaline, noradrenaline and dopamine)
- The adrenal gland is under the control of:
  - Pituitary adrenocorticotrophic hormone (ACTH) (steroid and androgen production)
  - Renal renin (aldosterone production)

Pathophysiology of the adrenal glands
Disorders of the adrenal glands include:
- Excess production of adrenal hormones, which result in different clinical entities:
  - Glucocorticoids: Cushing's syndrome
  - Mineralocorticoids: hyperaldosteronism
  - Androgens: adrenal tumours, congenital adrenal hyperplasia
  - Catecholamines: pheochromocytoma
- Hormonal undersecretion (adrenal failure)
  - Glucocorticoid and mineralocorticoid: Addison's disease
  - Lack of androgen and catecholamine production is not believed to have significant clinical manifestations

Endocrinology and Diabetes: Clinical Cases Uncovered. By R. Ajjan.
Published 2009 by Blackwell Publishing, ISBN: 978-1-4051-5726-1

- Adrenal disorders with no hormonal abnormality
  - Adrenal tumours

Investigation for adrenal dysfunction
Hormonal tests
- Static tests
  - Plasma renin activity, aldosterone, androgens (DHEA, testosterone), urinary catecholamines
- Suppressive tests
  - Dexamethasone suppression test
- Stimulating tests
  - Synacthen test

Imaging tests
- CT or MRI: can detect lesions >5 mm in diameter
- Ultrasound: can detect lesions >20 mm in diameter but can be technically difficult
- Venous sampling: can be used to investigate hormonal production by the glands, particularly in the presence of pathology in both adrenals (helps to differentiate unilateral from bilateral disease)

Full details of the above tests will be given under each disease entity (described below).

Overproduction of adrenal hormones
Glucocorticoid excess
Excessive secretion of glucocorticoid by an adrenal adenoma results in Cushing's syndrome with similar symptoms to ACTH-dependent Cushing's syndrome, except for the absence of pigmentation (because ACTH levels are suppressed). Causes of Cushing's syndrome are summarized in Table 14.

Clinical presentation
Onset is often insidious and symptoms may fluctuate. Patient presents with:
- Weight gain
- Central obesity with thin extremities
- Acne and hirsutism

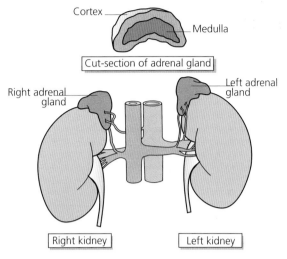

Figure 18 Anatomy of the adrenal glands.

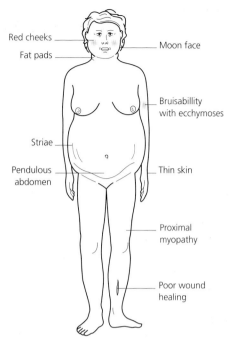

Figure 19 Clinical features of Cushing's syndrome (see text for full explanation).

Table 14 Causes of ACTH-dependent and ACTH-independent Cushing's syndrome.

ACTH-dependent Cushing's syndrome	ACTH-independent Cushing's syndrome
Pituitary tumour secreting ACTH (Cushing's disease)	Adrenal tumour secreting glucocortocoid (ACTH levels are suppressed)
Ectopic ACTH production (malignant tumours)	Long-term steroid treatment (respiratory disease, connective tissue disease)

- Easy bruising
- Low libido and menstrual irregularities
- Growth arrest in children
  Signs include (see Fig. 19)
- Facial appearance (moon-like face), with hirsutism and thinning of scalp hair
- Central obesity and abdominal striae
- Thin skin and evidence of bruising
- Proximal muscle weakness
- Hypertension
- Fractures (secondary to osteoporosis)
- Diabetes mellitus or impaired glucose tolerance
- Increased pigmentation does *not* occur in adrenal disease as ACTH levels are not increased (ACTH production is suppressed due to negative feedback)

Investigations
- Confirm the presence of excess cortisol
  ○ Midnight cortisol: in normal individuals, cortisol levels at midnight during sleep are undetectable. This test may be difficult to arrange as the patient needs to be admitted and a blood sample should be taken immediately after the patient is woken up at midnight (the patient should *not* be warned about having this test)
  ○ 24-h urinary cortisol: high levels are suggestive of the diagnosis
  ○ Overnight dexamethasone suppression test: give 0.5–1.0 mg of dexamethasone at 23:00 and measure cortisol at 09:00. Cortisol levels less than 50 nmol/L effectively rule out the diagnosis of Cushing's syndrome
  ○ Low-dose dexamethasone suppression test: give 0.5 mg dexamethasone ever 6 h for 2 days (eight doses) and check cortisol levels thereafter, which should be <50 nmol/L in the absence of Cushing's syndrome
- Differentiate between different causes of Cushing's syndrome
  ○ ACTH levels: these are suppressed in adrenal Cushing's but detectable in pituitary Cushing's disease or cases due to ectopic ACTH production

Table 15 Causes of increased aldosterone production.

Renin-dependent hyperaldosteronism (raised plasma renin activity)	Renin-independent hyperaldosteronism (suppressed plasma renin activity)
Renal hypoperfusion (renal artery stenosis, severe heart failure, cirrhosis)	Aldosterone-producing adrenal adenoma (Conn's syndrome) and rarely carcinoma
Renin-producing tumour (rare)	Bilateral adrenal hyperplasia

- High-dose dexamethasone suppression test: give 2 mg dexamethasone every 6 h for 2 days. If cortisol is suppressed to more than 50% of basal value, it suggests a diagnosis of pituitary Cushing's disease, ruling out the possibility of adrenal Cushing's syndrome
- Imaging
  - CT or MRI of the adrenal: shows a mass in adrenal Cushing's syndrome
  - Signs of malignant adrenal mass include: large size (>6 cm), heterogeneity (calcification and necrosis) and local invasion

Treatment
- Surgery for benign adrenal adenoma: prognosis is good
- Surgery followed by adrenolytic treatment (i.e. mitotane) for adrenal carcinoma: prognosis is poor as only one in five individuals survive for 5 years

Mineralocorticoid excess
This results from the increased production of aldosterone. Causes of increased aldosterone production are summarized in Table 15 (see also Fig. 20).

Box 9 Primary hyperaldosteronism

Primary hyperaldosteronism results in:
- Renal sodium retention
- Potassium and hydrogen ion loss
- Consequently leading to hypertension, hypokalaemia and metabolic alkalosis

---

Clinical presentation
- Often asymptomatic and diagnosis is made during investigation for hypertension
- Patients sometimes experience symptoms related to hypokalaemia such as muscle weakness and myopathy, and polyuria

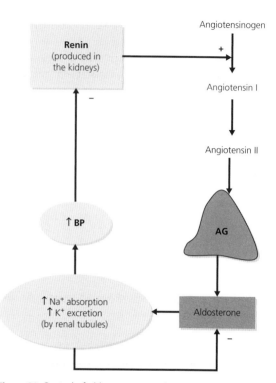

Figure 20 Control of aldosterone secretion. Decreased perfusion pressure in the kidneys results in renin secretion and the conversion of angiotensinogen to angiotensin I, and subsequently to angiotensin II (ATII) by angiotensin converting enzymes. ATII stimulates the adrenal glands to produce aldosterone, which increases sodium reabsorption and potassium excretion by the renal tubules. Increased plasma sodium results in water retention consequently raising the blood pressure and switching off renin secretion (negative feedback). Furthermore, low potassium has a negative feedback effect on aldosterone secretion. AG, adrenal gland; BP, blood pressure.

- Signs are moderately severe hypertension, particularly in a younger individual

Investigations
Hypertension with hypokalaemic alkalosis should be investigated for the possibility of hyperaldosteronism.
- Raised aldosterone/renin ratio is highly suggestive of the diagnosis
- Imaging
  - CT or MRI of the adrenals: differentiates between adrenal adenoma and bilateral hyperplasia
  - Adrenal vein sampling: reserved for difficult cases

Treatment
- For adrenal adenoma (Conn's syndrome), surgery is

the treatment of choice, which cures hypertension in two-thirds of cases
- For bilateral adrenal hyperplasia, the aldosterone antagonist, spironolactone or potassium-sparing diuretics, amiloride or triamterene, are used

Catecholamine excess

Adrenal medullary tumours (pheochromocytomas) can produce adrenaline and noradrenaline resulting in hypertension.

Clinical presentation

A pheochromocytoma should be suspected in:
- Severe or resistant hypertension
- Hypertension in the young
- Hypertension associated with the symptoms and signs summarized in Table 16

Symptoms are episodic and similar to how you feel when you are angry or before sitting an important exam.

Patients may present with a hypertensive crisis, which *can be fatal*. Factors precipitating a crisis include:
- Exercise
- Pressure on the abdomen (such as abdominal examination)

Table 16 Symptoms, signs and complications of pheochromocytomas.

Symptoms	Signs	Complications
Sweating	Hypertension	Cardiomyopathy
Pallor or flushing	Postural hypotension	Heart failure
Feeling of apprehension		Diabetes (rare)
Palpitations		Stroke
Throbbing headaches		

- Surgery
- Drugs
  - β-blocker (without previous α-blockade)
  - Anaesthetics
  - Opiates
  - Antidepressants

Pheochromocytomas can be part of a syndrome as shown in Table 17.

Investigations

- 24 h urine collection for catecholamines: due to the episodic nature of the disease, plasma levels of catecholamines can be normal and, therefore, measurement of these hormones in the urine is more reliable (two to three collections are necessary)
- Plasma catecholamines: this can be useful if samples are collected during a crisis
- Suppression tests (pentolinium or clonidine suppression): rarely needed to make a diagnosis
- Imaging
  - CT or MRI of adrenals: usually reveal a large adrenal tumour
  - Body MRI: if suspected extra-adrenal tumours
  - Meta-iodobenzylguanidine (MIBG) scan: can detect two-thirds of pheochromocytomas. Useful for investigating extra-adrenal tumours
- Adrenal venous sampling
  - Reserved for difficult cases
  - Presence of bilateral pathology

Treatment

- Surgery: removal of the tumour is curative
- Patient should be prepared before surgery with adequate α-blockade to avoid a hypertensive crisis, which may be fatal
- Medical treatment is not an option

The 'rule of 10' should be remembered when considering pheochromocytomas:

Table 17 Syndrome associated with pheochromocytomas (MEN, multiple endocrine neoplasia).

MEN II	Von-Hippel Lindau	Neurofibromatosis
Hyperparathyroidism	Cerebellar and retinal haemangioblastomas	Multiple neurofibromas
Thyroid carcinoma	Renal cell carcinoma	Café au lait spots
Pheochromocytoma (50%)	Pheochromocytoma (around 20%)	Pheochromocytoma (rare)

- 10% are malignant
- 10% are extra-adrenal (arising in the sympathetic or parasympathetic chain)
- 10% are familial (in which case screening should be preformed)

Adrenal failure

- Primary adrenal failure results in glucocorticoid and mineralocorticoid deficiency (commonly described as Addison's disease)
- Secondary adrenal failure results in glucocorticoid deficiency only

Causes of adrenal failure are summarized in Table 18.

Table 18 Causes of adrenal failure.

Primary adrenal insufficiency	Secondary adrenal insufficiency
Autoimmune (main cause in the Western world)	Autoimmune disease: autoimmune hypophysitis, isolated ACTH deficiency
Infiltrative disease: haemochromatosis, amyloidosis	Infiltrative disease: sarcoidosis, histiocytosis, haemochromatosis
Infections: tuberculosis, fungal infections, opportunistic infections (seen in patients with AIDS)	Infections: tuberculosis, pituitary abscess
Vascular	Vascular
Haemorrhage (anticoagulant therapy, meningococcal septicaemia)	Haemorrhage
Infarction	Infarction
Adrenoleucodystrophy: an inherited disease, associated with quadriplegia	Radiotherapy
Congenital adrenal hyperplasia	Head trauma
Drug induced	Drug induced
Ketoconazole (↓ cortisol synthesis)	Long-term steroid treatment results in suppression of ACTH production
Rifampicin (↑ cortisol metabolism)	
Malignant disease with adrenal metastasis	

Clinical presentation

- In glucocorticoid deficiency, presentation is similar to that described under pituitary failure except for the presence of pigmentation (secondary to high ACTH) and this can be seen in:
  - Palmar creases
  - Scar tissue
  - Buccal mucosa
- Aldosterone deficiency, resulting in:
  - Postural hypotension
  - Hyponatraemia
  - Hyperkalaemia
  - Metabolic acidosis

Isolated aldosterone deficiency may be secondary to impaired renin secretion (hyporeninaemic hypoaldosteronism). This is also known as renal tubular acidosis type IV, which can be seen in renal disease (such as diabetic nephropathy), and it is a condition that is probably underdiagnosed.

Investigations

- Disease should be suspected in the presence of:
  - Hypotension
  - Hyponatraemia
  - Hypokalaemic acidosis
- Random serum cortisol
  - Undetectable cortisol is diagnostic of adrenal insufficiency
- ACTH stimulation test (commonly known as synacthen test)
  - Failure of cortisol to rise after ACTH stimulation is diagnostic of adrenal insufficiency
- Renin and aldosterone
  - Aldosterone levels are low and renin levels are elevated in primary adrenal insufficiency
- Establish the cause
  - Adrenal autoantibodies
  - Adrenal imaging

Treatment

Emergency treatment is required in anyone with suspected adrenal insufficiency.

- Acute treatment
  - Intravenous hydrocortisone
  - Intravenous fluid
  - Watch for hypoglycaemia and correct as necessary
- Chronic treatment
  - Oral hydrocortisone given in two to three daily doses (to replace glucocorticoids)

○ Oral fludrocortisone (to replace mineralo-corticoids)

○ Treatment is monitored clinically and by measurement of electrolytes and plasma renin levels

• Patient education: all patients should be warned to double the dose of glucocorticoid in mild intercurrent illness and to give parenteral treatment in severe illness or prior to major surgery

Adrenal tumours

Adrenal tumours can be picked up during routine investigations for non-adrenal disease and these are often called 'incidentalomas'.

Box 10 Investigation of adrenal tumours

Any adrenal tumour should be investigated for the possibility of:

• Glucocorticoid production (i.e. Cushing's syndrome)
   ○ Cortisol suppression tests
• Mineralocorticoid production (i.e. Conn's syndrome)
   ○ High aldosterone/renin ratio
• Catecholamine production (i.e. pheochromocytoma)
   ○ High catecholamines on 24-h urine collection
• Androgen production (i.e. androgen-secreting tumours)
• High plasma androgen levels

Adrenal tumours may be non-functional (do not produce any hormones) and these can be simply followed up by repeated scanning. Adrenalectomy is advised for:

• Large tumours (>4 cm)
• Tumours with fast growth

(Large and fast growing tumours are more likely to be malignant.)

Congenital adrenal hyperplasia (CAH)

Congenital adrenal hyperplasia is an inherited disease characterized by a deficiency of one of the enzymes involved in cortisol biosynthesis (fully discussed in the reproductive section). The commonest is due to 21α-hydroxylase deficiency, which results in:

• Failure of cortisol and aldosterone synthesis
• Increased production of 17-OH-progesterone and testosterone

The clinical spectrum is very wide and includes:

• In severe cases (severe deficiency)
   ○ Salt wasting in the neonatal period (male or female).
   ○ Virilization of female fetus (affected female subjects are sometimes raised as males)
• Less severe cases (mild deficiency), these are usually clinically evident in females:
   ○ Hirsutism
   ○ Acne
   ○ Menstrual irregularities
   ○ Infertility

Investigations

High levels of hormones upstream of the enzymatic defect (elevated 17-OH-progesterone levels).

Treatment

• Cortisol replacement to suppress ACTH production, thereby limiting androgen production. Response to therapy is monitored:
   ○ Clinically
   ○ By assessing 17-OH-progesterone levels (aim to suppress to around twofold of normal)
• Fludrocortisone in severe cases with salt wasting. Response to therapy is monitored:
   ○ Clinically
   ○ Renin levels (aim to suppress into the normal range)

The reproductive system

Anatomy

The reproductive endocrine organs include the ovaries in females and testes in males.

- The ovaries are situated in the pelvis on either side of the uterus as shown in Fig. 21.
- During reproductive life, the ovaries contain follicles (each containing an oocyte) at different stage of maturation embedded in the ovarian stroma
- In adults, the testes are found in the scrotum, except in a minority with testicular mal descent, in which case the testicles can be in the inguinal canal
- In an adult male the testicular size is 15–25 ml (Fig. 22)
- Testes are composed of:
  - Interstitial or Leydig cells, which produce testosterone
  - Seminiferous tubules made up of germ (producing sperm) and sertoli cells (producing inhibin)

Full description of the female and male reproductive systems can be found in many other textbooks.

Physiology

- Ovaries have two functions
  - Endocrine: production of oestrogen and progesterone
  - Reproductive: storage and release of oocytes
- Testicles have two functions
  - Endocrine: production of testosterone
  - Reproductive: production of sperms

This section will mainly concentrate on the endocrine function of these organs.

Physiology of the female reproductive system

- Ovarian function is under the control of the hypothalamic-pituitary axis (Fig. 23)

- The hypothalamus produces gonadotrophin releasing hormones (GnRH) in a pulsatile fashion
- GnRH stimulate the pituitary to release follicle stimulating hormone (FSH) and luteinizing hormone (LH)
- FSH results in:
  - Growth and maturation of ovarian follicles (which contain the oocyte)
  - Stimulation of oestrogen production by follicular cells
- LH results in:
  - Ovulation (a surge in LH production is responsible for ovulation)
  - Maintenance of progesterone production by the corpus luteum
- Inhibin, secreted by the ovaries and under FSH control, has a negative feedback effect on FSH production
- Oestradiol has a negative feedback effect on FSH production but has a positive effect on LH surge (necessary for ovulation)

Box 11 The menstrual cycle

The menstrual cycle can be divided into:

- Follicular phase (day 6–13): around 20 follicles (each containing an oocyte) grow under the influence of FSH and secrete oestradiol
- Ovulation (day 14): a surge in LH results in ovulation (one oocyte is passed into the fallopian tubes)
- Luteal phase (day 15–25): after ovulation the corpus luteum forms from theca interna cells, which produce progesterone
- Premenstrual phase (day 25–28): LH levels fall, and theca cells lose the ability to maintain adequate progesterone production
- Menstruation (day 1–6): low progesterone levels lead to loss of endometrial support, which starts shedding and menstruation takes place

---

Endocrinology and Diabetes: Clinical Cases Uncovered. By R. Ajjan. Published 2009 by Blackwell Publishing, ISBN: 978-1-4051-5726-1

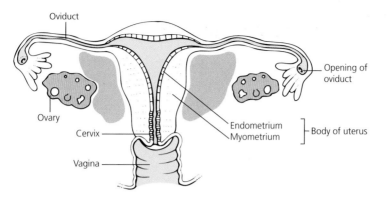

Figure 21 Anatomy and histology of the ovaries. Relationship of ovaries to the uterus and fallopian tubes. From Holt, RIG & Hanley, NA (2007) *Essential Endocrinology and Diabetes*, 5th edition. Blackwell Publishing, Oxford.

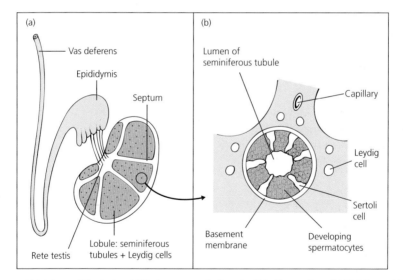

Figure 22 Anatomy and histology of the testes. (a) Testes are usually found within the scrotum. (b) Histology of the testes showing the seminiferous tubules, within which sertoli cells can be found. Leydig cells are found in the interstitial space. From Holt, RIG & Hanley, NA (2007) *Essential Endocrinology and Diabetes*, 5th edition. Blackwell Publishing, Oxford.

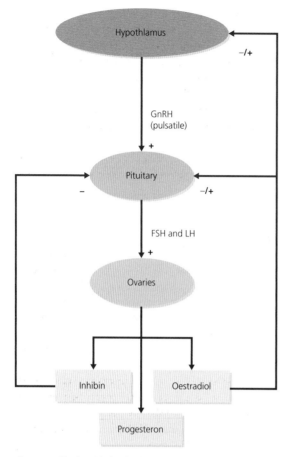

Figure 23 The hypothalamic-pituitary-ovarian axis. Gonadotrophin (GnRH), secreted in pulsatile fashion, stimulate follicle stimulating hormone (FSH) and luteinizing hormone (LH) production by the pituitary. FSH results in follicular growth and maturation in the ovary associated with oestradiol production. LH results in ovulation and subsequently maintains progesterone production by corpus luteum theca cells. Inhibin secretion by the ovaries, stimulated by FSH, has a negative feedback effect on pituitary FSH production. Oestradiol has a negative feedback effect on FSH production but it facilitates the LH surge necessary for ovulation.

- Effects of hormonal changes on the uterine endometrium include:
  - Repair and proliferation of the endometrium (oestradiol)
  - Increase endometrial thickness and preparation for implantation (progesterone)

Physiology of the male reproductive system
- Similarly to the ovaries, testicular function is under the control of the hypothalamic-pituitary axis (Fig. 24)

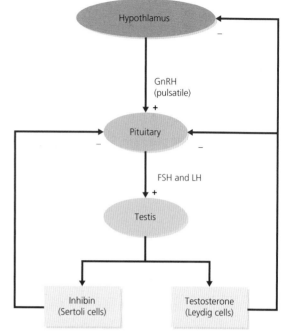

Figure 24 The hypothalamic-pituitary-testicular axis. Gonadotrophin (GnRH) secreted in pulsatile fashion, stimulates FSH and LH production by the pituitary. FSH is responsible for sperm maturation and also controls inhibin production. LH stimulates testosterone secretion by Leydig cells. Inhibin has a negative feedback effect on FSH production, whereas testosterone mainly suppresses LH production.

- Hypothalamic GnRH, secreted in pulses, regulate FSH and LH secretion by the pituitary
- FSH is important for sperm maturation
- LH is important for testosterone production by Leydig cells
- Inhibin, produced by sertoli testicular cells and under FSH control, has a negative feedback effect on FSH production
- Testosterone has a negative feedback effect, which mainly affects LH production

Pathophysiology of the endocrine reproductive system
Abnormalities of the female reproductive system:
- Menstrual abnormalities
- Premature ovarian failure
- Polycystic ovary syndrome (PCOS)
- Congenital adrenal hyperplasia
- Virilizing tumours

- Infertility
Abnormalities of the male reproductive system:
- Hypogonadism
- Gynaecomastia
- Testicular tumours
- Infertility

Menstrual abnormalities

This topic is covered in detail in other textbooks and is only briefly discussed here. Menstrual abnormalities can be divided into:

Physiological
- Prepubertal
- Pregnancy
- Lactation
- Menopause

Pathological

Primary amenorrhoea: the failure to reach menarche by the age of 16. This may be due to:
- Structural abnormality (such as imperforated hymen, congenital absence of the uterus)
- Genetic disorders (such as Turner's syndrome)
- Testicular feminization syndrome: the individual is genetically a male (XY chromosome) but phenotypically a female due to tissue insensitivity to androgens
- Causes of secondary amenorrhoea (see below)

Secondary amenorrhoea: the cessation of menstrual periods in women who had previously menstruated. Causes include:
- Ovarian, e.g. polycystic ovary disease, or premature ovarian failure due to a chromosomal abnormality (Turner's syndrome), autoimmune disease or iatrogenic cause (chemo- or radiotherapy, e.g. after cancer treatment)
- Uterine or fallopian tubes, e.g. adhesion in the uterus/fallopian tubes or uterine tumours
- Pituitary, e.g. hypopituitarism or prolactinoma
- Hypothalamic, e.g. excessive exercise (such as professional athletes), severe weight loss, stress (physical or psychological), hypothalamic tumours or infiltrative lesions
- General endocrine, these are usually associated with menstrual irregularities rather than amenorrhoea and include thyroid dysfunction and Cushing's syndrome

Clinical presentation

The patient presents with amenorrhoea or menstrual irregularities. It is important to establish in the history:

- Rule out physiological causes
- Establish growth and development of the child (particularly in primary amenorrhoea)
- Details of previous menstrual cycle (if any)
- Any recent stress/weight loss
- Past or present illness
- History of radiation or chemotherapy
- Previous pelvic operation or pelvic inflammatory disease
- Review drug history as some medications can cause amenorrhoea, e.g. previous use of oral contraceptive pills
- Presence of galactorrhoea

Investigations

Only hormonal investigations will be listed here. These include plasma levels of oestradiol, FSH, LH and prolactin and sex hormone binding globulin (SHBG).
- Low ovarian hormones and raised FSH/LH indicates primary ovarian failure (menopause or premature ovarian failure)
- Low ovarian hormones with low FSH/LH indicates pituitary or hypothalamic disease
- Prolactin should always be checked as raised levels result in suppression of GnRH production and subsequent menstrual irregularities (see pituitary section)
- Thyroid and/or adrenal abnormalities should be excluded in suspicious cases
- Karyotype in suspected conditions: Turner's syndrome (XO), testicular feminizing syndrome (XY)

Treatment
- Treat the cause
- Hormone replacement therapy should be considered in those with irreversible disease

Premature ovarian failure

This is defined as the development of menopause (low oestrogen and raised gonadotrophins) before the age of 40. Causes include:
- Chromosomal abnormalities: Turner's syndrome
  - The commonest X chromosome abnormality in females affecting 1 in 2500
  - There is a complete or partial absence of one X chromosome
  - Characteristic phenotype (Fig. 25, colour plate section) comprises short stature, webbed neck, widely spaced nipples and poor breast development, cubitus valgus and shortened metacarpals

○ Associated clinical abnormalities include aortic coarctation, left-sided heart defects, hypothyroidism and lymphoedema
- Autoimmune disease of the ovary
  ○ Can be associated with other organ-specific autoimmune disease (thyroid, type 1 diabetes, etc.)
- Iatrogenic
  ○ Chemotherapy
  ○ Radiotherapy
- Infections
  ○ Human immunodeficiency virus (HIV)
  ○ Mumps

Clinical presentation
- Subjects present before the age of 40 with oligo- or amenorrhoea
- Symptoms of oestrogen deficiency
  ○ Hot flushes
  ○ Mood swings
  ○ Fatigue
  ○ Dyspareunia

Investigations
- The combination of low oestradiol and high FSH/LH confirms the diagnosis
- Tests should be undertaken to investigate the cause as appropriate
  ○ Karyotype
  ○ Pelvic imaging

Complications
- Osteoporosis
- Increased risk of cardiovascular disease

Treatment
- Hormone replacement therapy

Polycystic ovary syndrome (PCOS)
- A very common condition
- The leading cause of hirsutism in women
- Characterized by:
  ○ Insulin resistance
  ○ Hyperandrogenaemia and low sex hormone binding globulin (SHBG) (hence, high levels of free testosterone)
  ○ Polycystic ovaries in the majority of cases
  ○ Failure of ovulation
  ○ Most patients are overweight

Clinical presentation
- Hirsutism
  ○ Face, abdomen, back and extremities
  ○ 95% of women presenting to the outpatient clinic with hirsutism have PCOS
  ○ Symptoms often begin around puberty
- Oligo- or amenorrhoea: secondary to unovulation
- Obesity: the majority of these patients are overweight
- Complications
  ○ Infertility
  ○ Endometrial carcinoma: absence of menstruation and regular shedding of the endometrium predisposes to endometrial carcinoma

Investigations
- Plasma levels of the following hormones should be checked:
  ○ Testosterone: usually raised
  ○ Sex hormone binding globulin: usually low
  ○ LH/FSH ratio: raised in two-thirds of patients
- Imaging
  ○ Ultrasound of the ovaries shows multiple cysts in the stroma in the majority of subjects (Fig. 26)
  ○ Measurement of endometrial thickness is also useful, which demonstrates endometrial hyperplasia
- Other tests: due to the association with insulin resistance patients should be screened for:
  ○ Diabetes
  ○ Lipid abnormalities

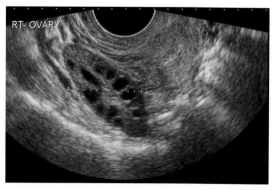

Figure 26 Ultrasound of the ovaries showing multiple cysts, a characteristic finding in polycystic ovary syndrome. Courtesy of Professor S. Atkin.

Treatment

These are a number of different treatments, which are summarized in Table 19.

- Weight loss: this reduces insulin resistance and, consequently, hyperandrogenaemia
- Suppression of ovarian androgen production
  - Oral contraceptive pills suppress FSH/LH production, and increase SHBG and thus reduce free testosterone levels

Table 19 Summary of treatment options for polycystic ovary syndrome.

Agent	Mode of action
Oral contraceptive pills	Suppression of ovarian stimulation
	Increase in sex hormone binding globulin
Spironolactone	Anti-androgen
Cyproterone acetate	
Flutamide	
Finasteride	
Metformin	Insulin sensitizers
Thiazolidinedione	
Clomiphene	Induction of ovulation
Gonadotrophins	(Fertility treatment)
Surgery	
Epilators, electrolysis, laser therapy	Cosmetic measures

- Anti-androgen agents
  - Androgen receptor blockers such as spironolactone, cyproterone acetate and flutamide (the latter rarely used due to risk of hepatic toxicity)
  - 5α-reductase inhibitors such as finasteride, which blocks the conversion of testosterone to its more potent androgen, dehydrotestosterone
- Insulin sensitizers
  - Metformin: can be helpful in some patients and may induce ovulation
  - Thiazolidinediones (glitazones): generally inferior to metformin
- Local cosmetic treatment for hirsutism
  - Epilators
  - Creams
  - Electrolysis
  - Laser therapy
- Fertility treatment (to induce ovulation)
  - Clomiphene citrate
  - GnRH preparations
  - Laparoscopic ovarian surgery

Congenital adrenal hyperplasia

- An autosomal recessive condition, which results in a defect in one of the enzymes involved in the synthesis of steroid hormones (Fig. 27)
- The commonest is 21α-hydroxylase (90%) and less commonly 11β-hydoxylase (<10%). Other enzyme deficiencies are rare

21α-hydroxylase deficiency (see Fig. 27)

This leads to:

- Cortisol deficiency, which may cause an Addisonian crisis in severe cases

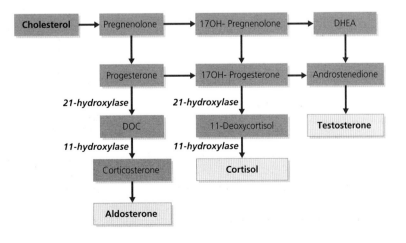

Figure 27 Synthesis of adrenal hormones. DHEA, dehydroepiandrosterone; DOC, deoxycorticosterone.

- Aldosterone deficiency, resulting in salt loss and hypotension
- Loss of negative feedback on the pituitary results in increased ACTH secretion and excessive production of 17-OH-progesterone, subsequently resulting in increased testosterone production and virilization
- Severity of the disease varies and depends on whether the individual has complete or partial enzyme deficiency

11β-hydroxylase deficiency (see Fig. 27)

This leads to:
- Increased androgen production resulting in virilization
- Increased corticosterone (DOC) accumulation resulting in hypertension

Clinical presentation

Only the common 21α-hydroxylase deficiency will be discussed here, which can present in two forms:

Complete 21α-hydroxylase deficiency (classical CAH)
- Female
  - Virilization
  - Clitoromegaly
  - Labial fusion
  - Renal salt wasting, resulting in hypotension
- Males
  - Renal salt wasting
  - Reduced fertility due to suppression of gonadotrophin secretion secondary to high adrenal testosterone production

Partial 21α-hydroxylase deficiency (non-classical CAH)
- Female
  - Hirsutism
  - Acne
  - Menstrual abnormalities
  - Infertility
- Male
  - Usually asymptomatic

Investigations
- Raised testosterone plasma levels
- Raised 17-OH-progesterone plasma levels
- Elevated renin plasma levels (due to defective production of aldosterone)

- Elevated ACTH plasma levels (due to defective cortisol production)
- Hormonal abnormalities can be minimal in non-classical CAH and, therefore, ACTH stimulation test may be required to make the diagnosis (raised 17-OH-progesterone after synacthen test)

Treatment
- Steroid treatment: this results in ACTH suppression and subsequently reduction in adrenal androgen production
- Fludrocortisone may be required in those with high renin levels
- Bilateral adrenalectomy in subjects with severe virilization

Virilizing tumours

These include tumours of the ovaries or adrenal glands, which can be benign or malignant.

Clinical presentation

Adrenal or ovarian virilizing tumours should be suspected in:
- Rapid onset of symptoms and signs of hyperandrogenism
- Virilization (severe hyperandrogenism), manifested as:
  - Clitoromegaly
  - Increased muscle mass
  - Deepening of voice
  - Frontal balding
- Symptoms related to the tumour
  - Abdominal mass
  - Ascites

Investigations
- Testosterone levels are usually very high
  - Imaging of adrenal/pelvis
  - Ultrasound
  - CT or MRI scan

Treatment
- Surgery
- Prognosis
  - In benign disease: excellent
  - In malignant disease: generally poor with 20–40% 5-year survival

Male hypogonadism

Defined as the failure of the testes to produce spermatozoa and/or testosterone. Causes of male hypogonadism include:

Primary

- Kleinefelter's syndrome (hypergonadotrophic hypogonadism)
  - Occurs in 1:500 births
  - Sex chromosome abnormality (47 chromosomes XXY)
  - Individuals are usually tall
  - Gynecomastia is common with increased risk of breast cancer
  - Intellectual dysfunction is found in around half the individuals
- Crytorchidism: failure of testes to migrate into the scrotum (undescended testes)
- Orchitis (testicular inflammation)
- Previous chemotherapy or radiotherapy
- Testicular trauma
- Alcohol excess
- Chronic illness

Secondary

- Hypothalamic
  - Hypothalamic tumours or infiltrative disease
  - Kallman's syndrome: a genetic disease characterized by hypogonadotrophic hypogonadism and anosmia (impaired sense of smell) in the majority
  - Idiopathic hypogonadotrophic hypogonadism: similar in presentation to Kallman's syndrome but sense of smell is intact
  - Severe exercise
  - Severe weight loss
  - Stress (physical or emotional)
  - Systemic illness
- Pituitary
  - Tumours
  - Infarct
  - Infiltrative disease

Clinical presentation

- Failure of progression through puberty
- Infertility
  - Sexual dysfunction (unable to maintain or absence of erection)
- Symptoms related to testosterone deficiency
  - Hot flushes
  - Tiredness
  - Decreased facial and/or body hair
  - Reduced libido
- The following can be found on examination:
  - Increased height: low testosterone in childhood results in delayed closure of epiphysis
  - Decreased facial and/or body hair
  - Small penis (usually in prepubertal disease)
  - Small testes
  - Anosmia
  - Gynaecomastia (discussed below)
  - Evidence of chronic disease (liver, renal, etc.)
- It should be noted that clinical presentation depends on:
  - Severity (partial or complete)
  - Age of onset
  - Duration of sex hormone deficiency

Investigations

- Testosterone, FSH, LH and prolactin should be checked
- Low testosterone with elevated FSH and LH indicates primary hypogonadism
- Low testosterone with low/normal FSH and LH indicates secondary hypogonadism
- Normal levels of testosterone/FSH/LH and prolactin usually rule out hypogonadism secondary to endocrine abnormality
- Sex hormone binding globulins are usually requested to enable calculation of free testosterone index, which gives a more accurate measurement of functional or active testosterone hormone levels

Treatment

- Treat the cause
- In cases of irreversible disease:
  - Testosterone replacement: transdermally, testosterone (as a gel) can be applied to the skin once a day; or by injections, these can be given every few weeks and with the newer preparations every few months
  - In cases of secondary irreversible gonadal failure, treatment with GnRH is a possibility in order to restore fertility

Gynaecomastia

Enlargement of the male breast is a relatively common condition. Causes include:

- Physiological
  - Puberty
  - Familial
- Drugs
  - Digoxin
  - Oestrogens
  - Spironolactone
  - Opiates
  - Antipsychotics
  - Heroin
  - Alcohol
- Hypogonadism (any cause, see above)
- Oestrogen or androgen producing tumours
- Chronic illness
  - Liver cirrhosis
  - Renal failure
- Breast cancer

Clinical presentation

- Patient presents with breast enlargement. Particular care should be taken in:
  - Rapid growth
  - Associated pain or tenderness
- Hypogonadal symptoms (see above)
- Drug history is essential (including recreational drugs)
- Examination
  - Palpate the breast: universal enlargement, lump, look for galactorrhoea
  - Palpate the testicles: rule out tumour and measure testicular size
  - Look for evidence of systemic illness

Investigations

- Blood tests
  - Testosterone
  - Oestradiol
  - FSH/LH
  - Prolactin
  - Human chorionic gonadotrophin (hCG, raised in some malignant tumours)
  - Liver, renal and thyroid function
- Imaging
  - Breast mammography if tumour is suspected
  - Testicular ultrasound
  - CT abdomen if adrenal lesion is suspected
- Biopsy
  - Breast tissue biopsy if tumour is suspected

Treatment

- Treat the underlying cause
- Surgical treatment in severe cases (reduction mammoplasty)

Infertility

Failure of pregnancy after 1 year of regular unprotected sex is defined as infertility. This can be very complicated to investigate.

Box 12 Causes of infertility

Causes of female infertility
- Hypothalamic abnormality
  - Hypothalamic amenorrhoea is commonly found in young athletes who undergo rigorous exercise
  - Kallman's syndrome
- Pituitary abnormality affecting gonadotrophin secretion
  - Pituitary tumours
  - Infiltrative disease
- Primary gonadal failure/abnormality
  - PCOS
  - Turner's syndrome
  - Primary ovarian failure
  - Chemotherapy or radiotherapy
- Tubular lesions
  - Adhesions due to previous infections
  - Endometriosis
- Uterine abnormalities
  - Congenital abnormalities
  - Adhesions due to previous infection
  - Fibroids
- Systemic debilitating disease

Causes of male infertility include:
- Hypothalamic disease
- Pituitary disease
- Testicular abnormality

Investigations

This is done in specialized centres. Briefly:

Male partner

Semen analysis
- Normal: investigate female partner
- Abnormal
  - Endocrine tests: normal testosterone, FSH, LH and prolactin usually rules out an endocrine cause; low

testosterone with high LH indicates primary gonadal failure; low testosterone with low/normal LH suggests secondary hypogonadism
- karyotyping in suspected Kleinfelter's syndrome
- Testicular ultrasound may show features of inflammation or testicular tumour

Female partner
- Endocrine tests
  - Normal testosterone, oestradiol, FSH, LH, TFTs and prolactin makes an endocrine cause for the infertility unlikely
  - Abnormalities with the above hormones should be investigated as discussed earlier
- Investigate for structural tubular and uterine abnormalities

Treatment
- Treat the cause
- Ovulation induction
- In some cases no cause for infertility is found and intrauterine insemination (IUI) or IVF may be considered

Puberty
- Average age of onset in girls is 10–12 years and boys 12–13 years
- Puberty involves breast development (the first sign), appearance of pubic hair and menarche in girls, whereas in boys it includes testicular and penile enlargement, appearance of pubic hair, voice change and increase in facial hair
- Puberty has five different stages (Tanner's stages) in girls and boys with specific measures applied to the parameters outlined above

Precocious puberty
- Onset of puberty before the age of 8 in girls and 9 in boys. Causes include:
  - Familial or idiopathic
  - Intracranial tumours
  - Rare genetic defects resulting in sex hormone production independent of central control

Delayed puberty
- Failure to progress to puberty after the age of 14 in girls and 16 in boys. Causes include:
  - Constitutional delay: fortunately the commonest cause
  - Chronic disease during the childhood period
  - Hypergonadotrophic hypogonadism: Kleinfelter's syndrome and Turner's syndrome
  - Hypogonadotrophic hypogonadism: Kallman's syndrome and disorders of the hypothalamus and pituitary

Investigations
- Blood tests
  - Testosterone
  - Oestradiol
  - FSH/LH
  - Prolactin
  - Karyotype
- Imaging of:
  - Ovaries
  - Testes
  - Pituitary/hypothalamus

Treatment
- Treat the cause

The pancreas

Anatomy

- The pancreas is situated behind the posterior wall of the abdomen (Fig. 28)
- It can be divided into:
  - Head: located within the duodenal curve
  - Body connected to the head through a slight constriction (neck)
  - Tail representing tapering of the body as it extends to the left approaching the gastric surface of the spleen
- The anterior surface of the pancreas is covered by the stomach, whereas the posterior surface is in contact with the large vessels (aorta, inferior vena cava and renal vessels)

Physiology

The pancreas has an:

- Exocrine function: secretes hormones into the gastrointestinal system to help with food digestion
  - This function of the pancreas is discussed in the gastroenterology book of this series
- Endocrine function: the pancreas is the main organ that regulates blood glucose levels.

Pathophysiology

- Defects in insulin secretion and action result in the development of diabetes mellitus
- Insulin deficiency is the pathophysiological abnormality in type 1 diabetes (T1DM)
- Insulin resistance with consequent β-cell dysfunction are the pathophysiological abnormalities in most cases of type 2 diabetes (T2DM)

Diabetes mellitus

- This common disease is characterized by raised blood glucose

Endocrinology and Diabetes: Clinical Cases Uncovered. By R. Ajjan.
Published 2009 by Blackwell Publishing, ISBN: 978-1-4051-5726-1

- Around 2–3 million individuals in the UK have diabetes but only half of them are diagnosed with the disease; in the rest the condition is clinically silent

Classification of diabetes

Type 1 diabetes (5–15% of cases)

- This is an autoimmune condition, resulting in destruction of pancreatic β-cells
- Subjects are often young (children or young adults) but the older age group can also be affected
- Latent autoimmune diabetes of adults (LADA) is also due to autoimmune β-cell destruction but the process is slower than classical T1DM and occurs in an older age group

---

Box 13 Cells responsible for the endocrine function of the pancreas

- β-cells, producing insulin:
  - Main hormone that maintains glucose homeostasis
  - Secretion is triggered by high plasma glucose
  - Composed of two polypeptide chains linked by disulphide bridges
  - Derived from proinsulin, which is packaged in the Golgi system of β-cells and transformed to the active form, insulin, by cleavage of C peptide by protease enzymes. Endogenous insulin production is associated with detectable C peptide levels in contrast to administering exogenous insulin, which can be useful in differentiating criminal or self-harm cases of insulin administration (raised insulin with undetectable C peptide levels) from endogenous insulin production (raised insulin and C peptide levels)
- α-cells, producing glucagons (discussed in the neuroendocrine section)
- δ-cells, producing somatostatin (discussed in the neuroendocrine section)
- PP cells, producing pancreatic polypeptide (discussed in the neuroendocrine section)

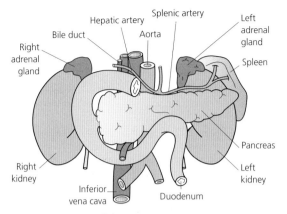

Figure 28 Anatomy of the pancreas.

Type 2 diabetes (75–85% of cases)

This is due to a combination of:

- Insulin resistance (usually as a result of obesity)
- β-cell dysfunction: insulin resistance is compensated for by an increase in insulin production by pancreatic β-cells. Eventually, these cells get 'worn out' and their insulin production decreases to a level that is unable to compensate for insulin resistance, leading to high plasma glucose and the development of diabetes

Type 2 diabetes is on the increase, mainly due to the increased prevalence of obesity and sedentary lifestyle

Secondary causes of diabetes (<5%)

- Pancreatic destruction
  - Pancreatitis
  - Trauma
  - Pancreatic cancer
  - Cystic fibrosis
  - Haemachromatosis (infiltration of the pancreas with iron)
- Endocrine disease
  - Acromegaly
  - Cushing's syndrome

Genetic defects (<5%)

Genetic defect in insulin secretion:

- Maturity onset diabetes of the young (MODY)
  - An autosomal dominant condition
  - A number of different types have been described, the commonest are due to mutation in genes for hepatic nuclear factor (HNF)1α, known as MODY 3, and glucokinase, known as MODY 2

- Mitochondrial mutations

Genetic defect in insulin action:

- Resulting in severe insulin resistance (very rare)

Drug induced (<5%)

- Glucocorticoid treatment: particularly in those receiving high dose of steroids
- Thiazides

Gestational diabetes (<5%)

- Diabetes that occurs during pregnancy
- Resolves spontaneously after giving birth
- Associated with increased risk of macrosomic (large) babies
- Affected women are at high lifetime risk of developing T2DM (up to one-third)

From the practical point of view, it is important to distinguish between type 1 and type 2 diabetes as failure to initiate insulin in a type 1 diabetes patient may result in death. This is fully discussed below.

Clinical presentation

There are a wide range of symptoms, including:

- Polyuria secondary to osmotic diuresis
- Polydipsia or increased thirst
- Visual disturbances: due to changes in the lens, secondary to high glucose levels
- Repeated skin infections
- Vaginal candidiasis (thrush) is common in female subjects
- Tiredness
- Weight loss (usually in type 1 diabetes)
- The patient may present with associated complications such as:
  - Myocardial infarction
  - Stroke
  - Renal disease
- In type 2 diabetes, the disease is commonly clinically silent and is discovered during investigations for other pathologies

During assessment of patients, it is important to differentiate T1DM from T2DM as management of these conditions is entirely different (see Table 20). The following should be taken into account:

- Detailed history: patients with T1DM present with short history of symptoms (days to weeks), in contrast to individuals with T2DM (months to years)
- The presence of weight loss, particularly in a younger individual, suggests T1DM

Table 20 Summary of the main features of type 1 diabetes (T1DM) and type 2 diabetes (T2DM).

	T1DM	T2DM
Aetiology	Autoimmune (β-cell destruction)	Insulin resistance and β-cell dysfunction
Peak age	12 years (can occur at any age)	60 years (increasingly seen at a young age due to obesity)
Prevalence	0.3%	Around 6%
Presentation	Osmotic symptoms (days to weeks), weight loss, DKA. Patient usually slim	Osmotic symptoms (months to years), diabetic complications. Patient usually obese
Treatment	Diet and insulin	Diet, exercise (weight loss), oral hypoglycaemic agents, insulin later

DKA, diabetic ketoacidosis.

• Individuals with T1DM tend to be thin (but not always) and those with T2DM tend to be overweight (but not always)
• Although rare, causes of secondary diabetes should be kept in mind and appropriate investigations should be arranged if necessary
• The presence of a family history suggestive of an autosomal dominant condition, particularly in those with diabetes at a young age, should alert to the possibility of MODY
• All patients (particularly older subjects) should be assessed for the presence of complications (macrovascular and microvascular complications, detailed below)

Complications of diabetes
Acute complications
Diabetic ketoacidosis (DKA)
• DKA is due to the absence of insulin and, therefore, it is mainly seen in patients with T1DM
• Not uncommonly, DKA is the first presentation of T1DM
• The absence of insulin results in switching from glucose to fat metabolism (in order to provide energy), a pathway that is associated with accumulation of ketone bodies, which cause metabolic acidosis
• Therefore, ketoacidosis is characterized by the presence of:
  ○ Acidosis (due to the accumulation of ketone bodies)
  ○ Dehydration (due to osmotic diuresis and vomiting, see below)

Diabetic hyperosmolar non-ketotic hyperglycaemia (HONK)
• A complication of T2DM, usually seen in the elderly
• Characterized by high glucose levels and severe dehydration
• Acidosis is usually absent

Hypoglycaemia
• This is discussed under the treatment of diabetes below

Chronic complications
Macrovascular (large vessel) complications
Patients with diabetes are at high risk of cardiovascular disease including:
• Ischaemic heart disease (IHD): all newly diagnosed diabetes patients should be assessed for the possibility of IHD
  ○ History: chest pain or shortness of breath on exertion
  ○ ECG: previous myocardial infarction, ischaemic changes
  ○ More sophisticated tests if in doubt (exercise test, angiogram)
• Cerebrovascular disease:
  ○ History of weakness or slurred speech should alert to the possibility of this diagnosis
  ○ Any neurological signs will warrant further investigations

- Peripheral vascular disease
  - History of pain in the legs on exertion
  - Feel the foot pulses

Microvascular (small vessel) complications

These include retinopathy, nephropathy and neuropathy.

- Retinopathy: the following changes can be observed:
  - Background changes (minor changes): microaneurysms, small intraretinal haemorrhages (dots) and hard exudates due to the leakage of lipids
  - Preproliferative changes (serious changes, need attention): soft exudates (areas of infarction), also known as cotton wool spots, and intraretinal microvascular abnormalities (IRMA), tortuous and dilated looking vessels occurring as a result of retinal ischemia
  - Proliferative changes (very serious changes, need immediate attention): new vessel formation
- Nephropathy
  - Microalbuminuria: excretion of small amounts of albumin in the urine. This is an early stage of diabetic nephropathy, which can be reversible
  - Macroalbuminuria: excretion of large amounts of albumin in the urine. This is seen in more advanced stages
  - Raised urea and creatinine: indicates renal failure
- Neuropathy
  - Peripheral: altered sensation in the feet, which predisposes to foot ulcers; Charcot's osteoarthropathy, results in bone fractures and deformity and can be difficult to diagnose and treat (Fig. 29, colour plate section); and neuropathy can also involve a main nerve or a group of nerves (third nerve palsy for example), causing sensory or motor abnormalities
  - Autonomic: can result in orthostatic hypotension, gastrointestinal symptoms (vomiting, diarrhoea), or erectile dysfunction

Investigations

1. Confirm the diagnosis of diabetes:
- Fasting plasma glucose
  - Levels above 7.0 mmol/L in the presence of symptoms or two tests above 7.0 mmol/L in the absence of symptoms confirm the diagnosis of diabetes
- Subjects with fasting glucose >6.0 but ≤7.0 mmol/L are labelled as having impaired fasting glucose and should undergo a glucose tolerance test (see below)

- Random plasma glucose
  - Levels above 11.0 mmol/L in the presence of symptoms confirm the diagnosis
- Oral glucose tolerance test
  - This should be performed in unclear cases
  - Subjects are given 75 g glucose and plasma glucose is assessed at 0 min and 120 min
  - Individuals with 2-h glucose <7.8 mmol/L: diabetes ruled out
  - Individuals with 2-h glucose >11.1 mmol/L: diabetes is confirmed
  - Individuals with 2-h glucose >7.8 and <11.1: impaired glucose tolerance is present (a prediabetic condition-risk of future diabetes is high)

2. Differentiate between types of diabetes
- A careful history is probably the most important tool to differentiate between different types of diabetes

---

Box 14 How to assess a newly diagnosed diabetes patient

Take a careful history
- Onset of symptoms: sudden (days/weeks) or gradual (months or years)
- Any history of weight loss
- Any family history
  - Autoimmunity: a personal or family history of autoimmunity (thyroid disease, vitiligo, coeliac disease, etc.), should raise the possibility of T1DM
  - Diabetes at a young age in an autosomal dominant fashion: should raise the possibility of MODY
- Check weight and body mass index (BMI): overweight subjects are more likely to have T2DM
- Look for signs of secondary diabetes (Cushing's syndrome, acromegaly, etc.)
- Check for the presence of complications (particularly in those with suspected T2DM)
  - Macrovascular: chest pain or breathlessness on exertion; history of cerebrovascular accident (CVA) or transient ischaemic attacks (TIA) (slurred speech, limb weakness); history of leg pain after exercise is suggestive of peripheral vascular disease; need to do a thorough cardiovascular examination
  - Microvascular: history of foot ulcers/swelling of the joints (examine the feet and check sensation using monofilament test); history of visual abnormalities (examine the fundi for diabetic retinopathy); renal disease is clinically silent in the early stages of the disease (check urine for microalbuminuria)

- Urine dipstick: this is an essential test in all diabetes patients. The presence of heavy ketonuria is indicative of T1DM. Ketonuria may also occur after prolonged fasting
- Laboratory tests can be useful in difficult cases:
  - Anti-glutamic acid decarboxylase (GAD) and anti-tyrosine phosphatase (IA-2) antibodies: antibodies against one or both molecules are present in around 80% of patients with T1DM. Their absence does not rule out the diagnosis of T1DM
  - Genetic testing: in suspected MODY commonest are mutations in HNF1α (MODY 3) and glucokinase (MODY 2) genes
  - Cases with suspected secondary cause: ferritin levels (haemachromatosis), CT abdomen in pancreatic cancer, Cushing's syndrome and acromegaly
3. Investigate for the presence of complications
- Acute
  - If in doubt whether the patient has early DKA, you can measure venous pH and bicarbonate (bicarbonate <15 mmol/L with or without low pH is diagnostic)
  - Do *not* miss the diagnosis of acute diabetic ketoacidosis, which may be fatal if not treated appropriately
- Chronic
  - ECG: this should be done in all newly diagnosed diabetes subjects as silent myocardial infarction is common in this group of patients
  - CT head and carotid Doppler: in case of history of TIA
  - Doppler of peripheral arteries: in case of history or examination suggesting peripheral vascular disease
  - Urinary microalbumin and U&Es to rule out nephropathy
  - Nerve conduction tests: in the presence of atypical neuropathic changes

Treatment
Treatment of type 1 diabetes (T1DM)
Patients with T1DM should be treated with insulin. There are different preparations of insulin, which are briefly discussed here. At present, the main insulin preparations in use are human insulin and insulin analogues. Animal insulin preparations (bovine and pork) are very rarely used these days.

Types of insulin:
- Human insulin preparations
  - Short (or fast) acting insulin (Actrapid): starts

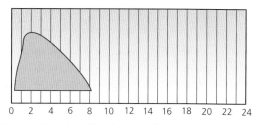

Figure 30 Duration of insulin cover after actrapid injection (h).

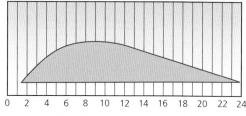

Figure 31 Duration of insulin cover after insulatard injection (h).

working in 30 min and peaks at 2–4 h after injection, covers up to 6–8 h post injection (Fig. 30)
  - Intermediate acting insulin or NPH insulin (Insulatard): starts working in 2 h and peaks 8 h post injection, covers for 16-20 h (Fig. 31)
  - Mixtures: short and intermediate acting with varied proportions; humulin M1 (10% short and 90% intermediate acting), humulin M3 (30% short and 70% intermediate acting) (Fig. 32)
- Analogue insulin preparations
  - Ultra-short (or ultra-fast) acting insulins (lispro, aspart, glulisine): start working almost immediately and peak at 1–2 h post injection and cover for around 4 h post injection
  - Long acting insulins (glargine, detemir): relatively flat profile (minimal peak, thus less chance of hypoglycaemia), start working in 2 h and last 20–24 h post injection
  - Mixtures: ultra-short acting analogues with intermediate insulin. There are no mixtures with long acting insulin analogues

How to give insulin injections
There are a number of regimes that can be used in T1DM but the most widely adopted are:
- Twice daily injections with mixture of insulins (i.e. Novomix 30, Humulin M3, Humalog mix 25) (Fig. 33)
- Four daily injections of insulin: also called basal bolus regime (Fig. 34)

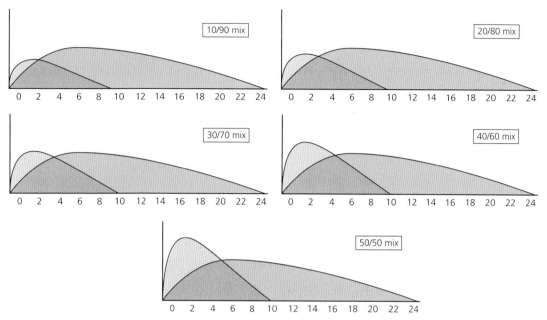

Figure 32 Duration of insulin cover after injection of different insulin mixtures (h).

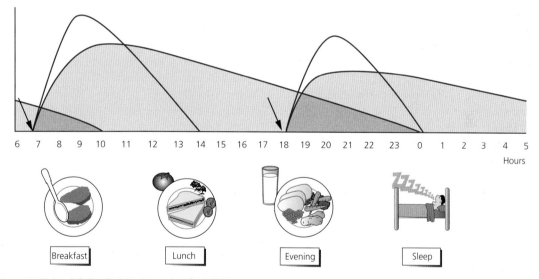

Figure 33 Twice daily insulin injection regime for T1DM.

○ One injection of intermediate or long acting insulin (to cover basal insulin)

○ Three injections of short acting or ultra-short acting insulin with meals (bolus insulin)

○ Basal bolus regime gives better flexibility and has a lower risk of hypoglycaemic episodes

In T2DM patients:

• Single injection of intermediate or long acting insulin can be added to existing oral hypoglycaemic agents

• Above regimes (same as T1DM) can also be used if one injection of insulin is not controlling plasma glucose levels

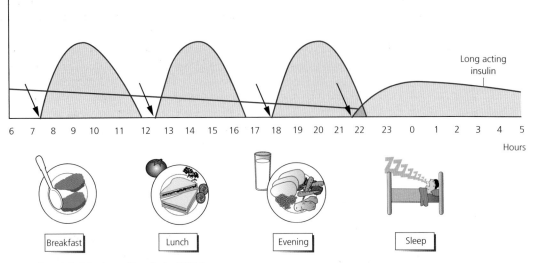

Figure 34 Four daily injections of insulin for T1DM.

How to start a newly diagnosed T1DM patient on insulin?

Newly diagnosed patients can be started on two or four injections of insulin after appropriate education, which is best done by the diabetes nurse specialist.

- Starting total 24-h dose of insulin is usually around 0.3–0.6 unit/kg, divided into:
  - Half to two-thirds of the dose as intermediate/long acting insulin
  - One-third to half the dose as short acting insulin
- A newly diagnosed patient weighing 70 kg can be started on:
  - Mixture of insulin 12 units morning and 8 units evening
  - Basal bolus: 8–10 units of intermediate/long acting and 2–6 units of fast/ultra-fast acting with meals
- It is good practice to teach insulin-treated patients carbohydrate counting (assessment of carbohydrate in each meal) to adjust the doses of insulin injections according to meal size

What are the complications of insulin treatment?

- Hypoglycaemia
  - All patients should be warned about the symptoms of hypoglycaemia, which can be very unpleasant including: tremor, sweating, nausea and feeling hungry
  - All patients should be properly educated to learn how to manage a hypoglycaemic episode (detailed below)
  - Lipoatrophy and lipohypertrophy at insulin injection sites: the former is rarely seen now but the latter can still occur (Fig. 35, colour plate section). Further injection into affected areas should be avoided

Other than daily injections, are there any other modes of delivery for insulin?

- Insulin can be delivered by an insulin pump, using a cannula placed in the abdomen (changed every 2–3 days)
  - Insulin is continuously infused with bolus doses given with meals
- Inhaled insulin
  - An insulin preparation, which can be given through inhalation. It only substitutes short acting insulin and the patient still needs to inject the long or intermediate acting insulin

What to do with a T1DM patient during clinic reviews?

- Assess diabetes control
  - Review blood glucose diary, paying particular attention to highs and troughs
  - Is there any particular pattern for the sugar readings? For example, high fasting sugar indicates the need for higher doses of intermediate or long acting insulin; high post meal sugars indicate the need for higher short acting insulin before the meal
  - Check HbA1c, which gives an indication of the average diabetes control over the previous 6 weeks

- Check for associated complications
  - Cardiovascular (particularly in older patients); check blood pressure in all patients
  - Nephropathy (check urine for albumin excretion)
  - Retinopathy (regular retinal examination or photography)
  - Foot examination: pulses and peripheral sensation

Treatment of type 2 diabetes (T2DM)
- Education of patients is very important
- The importance of diet and exercise should be emphasized
- All patients should be reviewed by a dietician for appropriate advice
- Measures to induce weight loss (most of these patients are overweight) should be encouraged/implemented
- In the initial phases of the disease diet and exercise may be enough to maintain good diabetes control
- Patients will eventually need medical intervention with oral hypoglycaemic agents or insulin

Oral hypoglycaemic agents
These have proliferated in the past decade or so and we now have a number of different treatment options. These include:
- Biguanides (main agent is metformin)
  - The first-line agent in obese T2DM patients
  - Metformin lowers blood glucose levels by: reducing hepatic glucose output (decrease in glycogenolysis), reducing glucose absorption and mildly reducing insulin resistance
  - Effective, cheap and safe
  - Use of this agent is associated with weight loss, which is welcome in subjects with diabetes
  - Side effects are mainly gastrointestinal (nausea, bloating) and these are minimized by a gradual increase in drug dose or use of long acting preparations
  - Contraindications include: renal failure – if creatinine is >150 μmol/L, the drug should be discontinued (or not started) due to fears of inducing lactic acidosis; advanced heart or liver failure – again there is a risk of inducing lactic acidosis. Use of metformin in mild heart failure or minor derangement of liver function is perfectly safe
- Insulin secretagogues
  - Sulphonylureas: gliclazide, glibenclamide and glimepiride are probably the most widely used agents

in the UK. These agents lower blood glucose by stimulating pancreatic insulin secretion. Side effects include hypoglycaemia and weight gain
  - Meglitinides: natiglinide and repaglinide are the most widely used agents. These increase insulin secretion by the pancreas, an effect that is more pronounced after a meal. They are less commonly associated with hypoglycaemia and weight gain compared with sulphonylureas. In practice, they are often less effective at reducing glucose levels compared with sulphonylureas
- Insulin sensitizers
  - Thiazolidinediones (also known as glitazones), pioglitazone and rosiglitazone, are stimulators of the peroxisome proliferators nuclear receptor (PPAR)-γ, which results in improvement in insulin resistance and decrease in blood sugar
  - These agents have cardiovascular protective features
  - Recent analysis, however, indicates that rosiglitazone has a neutral effect on cardiovascular events, whereas pioglitazone may reduce the risk
  - These agents can cause fluid retention and, therefore, they are contraindicated in subjects with heart failure
  - These agents induce weight gain
- Drugs that interfere with glucose absorption
  - α-Glucosidase inhibitors (acarbose is perhaps the most widely used agent in this group)
  - Use of these agents in the UK is limited due to a modest blood glucose lowering effect and gastrointestinal side effects, mainly bloating, which are very common
- Agents working on the glucagon-like peptide-1 (GLP-1) system
  - New agents introduced in the UK in 2007
  - GLP-1 is a natural hormone secreted by the gastrointestinal tract in response to meals
  - GLP-1 stimulates insulin secretion by the pancreas and inhibits glucagon production, thereby lowering plasma glucose levels
  - GLP-1 has a very short half-life as it is metabolized by dipeptidyl peptidase (DPP)-4 enzymes and quickly cleared from the circulation
- GLP-1 analogues (exenatide)
  - Work similarly to native GLP-1 but are slowly metabolized by DPP-4 enzymes, resulting in a longer half-life in the circulation

Table 21 The main features of the new hypoglycaemic agents, DPP-4 and glucagon-like peptide-1 (GLP-1) analogues.

	DPP-4	GLP-1 analogues
Administration	Oral	Injections
Efficacy	++	+++
Weight	Neutral	Weight loss
Side effects	Little	15–20% (gastrointestinal)

Table 22 Site and mechanism of action of the cannabinoid receptor blocker, rimonabant.

Site	Mechanism
Hypothalamus	Decreases appetite
Muscle	Increases glucose uptake
Gastrointestinal tract	Increases satiety signals

    ○ Injected s.c. twice a day resulting in a reduction in blood sugar levels and weight loss. Side effects including gastrointestinal symptoms in relatively large number of patients (around one-fifth), which may improve with continued use of the drug
• DPP-4 inhibitors (sitagliptine/vildagliptine)
    ○ Inhibition of DPP-4 results in slower breakdown of 'native' GLP-1 and consequently an increase in plasma levels
    ○ These agents are less effective at reducing blood glucose levels compared with GLP-1 analogues
    ○ DPP-4 inhibitors are weight neutral
    ○ They have advantages over GLP-1 analogues in that they are given orally (no injections are needed) and side effects are minimal
Table 21 summarizes the main characteristics of GLP-1 analogues and DPP-4 inhibitors.
• Slimming tablets
    ○ Orlistat inhibits intestinal lipase thereby reducing fat absorption. It is important to comply with a low-fat diet whilst on treatment with this agent, otherwise it may cause an oily (pretty unpleasant) diarrhoea
    ○ Sibutramine is central appetite suppressant, which may induce tachycardia and high blood pressure (regular monitoring is mandatory). This can be a problem in hypertensive patients with diabetes

    ○ Rimonabant is a new agent for weight reduction licensed for use in the UK in 2007. It is a cannabinoid receptor type 1 (CB1) blocker and works at multiple levels (see Table 22). It has a role in the management of multiple cardiometabolic factors, e.g. improvement in lipid profile, improvement in glycaemic control and reduction in central obesity. Side effects include depression in up to 15% of treated individuals, and, therefore, this agent is contraindicated in those with a history of depression or during treatment with antidepressants
The mode of action and contraindications of each of the antidiabetic agents is summarized in Fig. 36 and Table 23.

When do we need to move patients from oral hypoglycaemic treatment to insulin?

• Failure of oral hypoglycaemic agents to maintain adequate glucose levels (metformin is usually continued with insulin treatment)
• Pregnancy: insulin is safe to use during pregnancy and, therefore, pregnant women with diabetes are usually treated with insulin only
• Severe illness or operation requiring hospital admission: oral hypoglycaemic agents are temporarily stopped

Management of diabetic complications
Acute complications
Diabetic ketoacidosis

• A medical emergency with a death rate of 3–5%
• Is due to the lack of insulin and subsequent switch from glucose to fatty acid metabolism, which results in the production of ketone bodies:
    ○ Acetoacetic acid
    ○ Hydoxybutyric acid
    ○ Acetone (giving DKA patients acetone-smelling breath)
• Subjects with DKA have three fundamental abnormalities
    ○ Metabolic acidosis, which causes abdominal pain and vomiting, and compensatory hyperventilation (Kussmaul respiration): blowing off CO_2 results in respiratory alkalosis, trying to compensate for the metabolic acidosis
    ○ Dehydration, secondary to osmotic diuresis (high glucose levels) and vomiting
    ○ Electrolyte imbalance, including hyperkalaemia, secondary to metabolic acidosis, hyponatraemia and 'relative' hypokalaemia due to vomiting

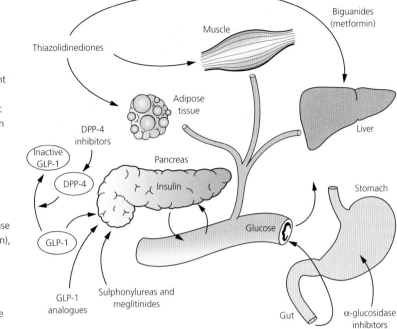

Figure 36 Mode of action of different oral hypoglycaemic agents. The biguanide metformin reduces hepatic glucose uptake and has a mild insulin sensitizing effect. Thiazolidinediones reduce insulin resistance, making insulin more effective at reducing blood sugar. Sulphonylureas and meglitinides stimulate pancreatic insulin secretion. GLP-1 analogues have a similar effect to GLP-1 (increase insulin and reduce glucagon secretion), but are slowly degraded by DPP-4 enzymes. DPP-4 inhibitors interfere with GLP-1 degradation resulting in increased levels of this hormone. α-Glucosidase inhibitors reduce glucose absorption.

PART 1: BASICS

Table 23 Main side effects and contraindications of agents used to control blood sugar levels in individuals with T2DM. Pregnant women with diabetes should be treated with insulin and oral hypoglycaemic agents are generally contraindicated.

Agent	Side effects	Contraindication
Metformin	Gastrointestinal (bloating, diarrhoea)	Renal failure (even if mild)
		Advanced heart and liver failure
		Pregnancy (relative contraindication)
Sulphonylureas	Hypoglycaemia	Pregnancy
	Weight gain	
Thiazolidinediones	Fluid retention	Heart failure
	Weight gain	Pregnancy
GLP-1 analogues	Gastrointestinal	Pregnancy
DPP-4 inhibitors	Rare	Pregnancy
Orlistat	Diarrhoea	Pregnancy
Sibutramine	Hypertension	Uncontrolled hypertension
	Tachycardia	Pregnancy
Rimonabant	Depression	History or current treatment of depression
		Pregnancy

- Causes of DKA:
  - New diagnosis of T1DM in 20% of cases
  - In a known diabetic patient, DKA can be due to: infection in 35% of cases, non-compliance with insulin injection in 30%, and errors in insulin administration and dose calculation in 15%. In older patients, DKA may be precipitated by an ischaemic event such as myocardial infarction

Clinical presentation of DKA

DKA subjects can present with a variety of symptoms:
- Gastrointestinal
  - Nausea
  - Vomiting
  - Abdominal pain
- Generally feeling unwell
- Coma in advanced cases
- In those with known diabetes, DKA should be suspected in anyone who is not feeling or looking well
- In subjects with suspected DKA who are not known to have diabetes, a proper history is paramount to make the correct diagnosis

Investigations in suspected DKA

These consist of:
- 1. Confirm the diagnosis
  - Raised glucose levels: glucose can be only slightly elevated
  - Reduced plasma bicarbonate levels with or without low pH (bicarbonate <15 mmol/L confirm the diagnosis of DKA)
  - Presence of ketonuria
- 2. Rule out precipitating cause:
  - Chest X-ray (? infection)
  - Check urine for the possibility of infection
  - ECG (? myocardial infarction)
  - Take blood and urine samples for culture
  - Note that a high white cell count may occur in subjects with DKA in the absence of infection

Treatment of DKA

This should be promptly started and consists of fluid and insulin replacement as well as management of electrolyte imbalance. In addition, treatment should be directed to the precipitating cause (if any). Monitoring of patients after initial treatment is very important and local hospital guidelines for the management of these patients should be strictly followed.

- Fluid
  - Fluid replacement usually starts with normal saline (0.9%): 1 L over the first h, 1 L over 2 h, then 1 L every 4–6 h, with careful monitoring of the patient and adjustment of fluid replacement accordingly. Normal saline should be substituted with 5% dextrose infusion once plasma glucose drops below 12–15 mmol/L (different protocols use different cut-offs)
- Potassium
  - Failure to replace potassium can result in severe hypokalaemia, which may cause cardiac arrhythmias, potentially resulting in death. Serum potassium is usually elevated on initial presentation due to the presence of acidosis, despite low total body potassium. Potassium levels quickly drop after initiation of DKA treatment, as both insulin replacement and correction of acidosis shift the potassium from the extracellular space into the cells. As a rough guide, 20 mmol/L potassium should be added to the fluid in patients with normokalaemia, 40 mmol/L to those with hypokalaemia and no potassium should be given to those with hyperkalaemia. Monitoring potassium levels (every 2–4 h) during treatment is extremely important
- Insulin
  - Insulin is started as an i.v. infusion at around 0.1 u/kg/h and adjusted according to a sliding scale insulin (see Table 24). Capillary glucose should be checked hourly and i.v. insulin should only be stopped once the urine is ketone-free and the patient is clinically well
- Bicarbonate
  - This is very rarely given; only in cases of severe acidosis not responding to conventional treatment. Bicarbonate administration should only be done in an intensive care setting and after the involvement of a senior colleague with expertise in DKA management

Table 24 An example of sliding scale insulin. This is only a guide and different sliding scales can be used as some individuals require higher doses of insulin whereas others need less.

Capillary glucose	Insulin dose
<4.0 mmol/L	0.5 units/h (with i.v. dextrose): review
4.1–10.0 mmol/L	2 unit/h
10.0–16.0 mmol/L	4 units/h
>16.0 mmol/L	6 units/h: review

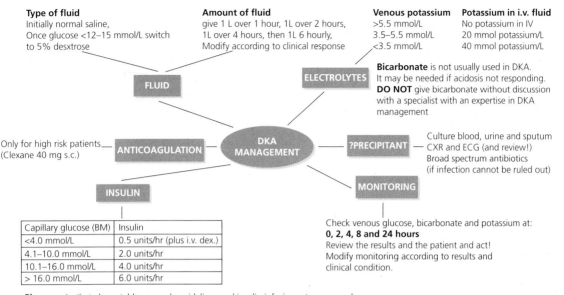

Capillary glucose (BM)	Insulin
<4.0 mmol/L	0.5 units/hr (plus i.v. dex.)
4.1–10.0 mmol/L	2.0 units/hr
10.1–16.0 mmol/L	4.0 units/hr
> 16.0 mmol/L	6.0 units/hr

Please note that above tables are only guidelines and insulin infusion rate may need modification. **Continue i.v. insulin/dextrose until urine is ketone-free.**

Figure 37 Summary of the management of diabetic ketoacidosis.

- Precipitating cause(s)
  ○ Around two-thirds of DKA cases are due to newly diagnosed type 1 diabetes or compliance problems/errors in insulin administration in known diabetic patients. In around one-third, DKA is due to other causes such as infection or myocardial infarction and these conditions should be treated appropriately
- Other measures
  ○ Some recommend low-dose heparin to prevent thromboembolism, but there is no clear evidence to support this practice, which is perhaps unnecessary unless other risk factors exist (prolonged immobility)
  ○ A nasogastric tube may need to be inserted in those with severe vomiting or in those with impaired conscious level
- Monitoring
  ○ Capillary glucose should be checked hourly and blood samples should be taken every 2–4 h for U&Es, bicarbonate and venous glucose. The clinical condition of the patient should be regularly assessed
  The management of DKA is summarized in Fig. 37.

Hyperosmolar non-ketotic hyperglycaemia (HONK)
- This is characterized by the gradual development of hyperglycaemia

- Mortality is very high approaching 50% in these patients
- Causes include:
  ○ Omission of oral hypoglycaemic agents or insulin (rarely it can be the first presentation of T2DM)
  ○ Infection
  ○ Vascular events such as myocardial infarction and stroke

Clinical presentation of HONK
- Insidious onset of symptoms with ill health for weeks
- History of osmotic symptoms
- Symptoms of precipitating cause
- Coma

Investigations in HONK
- Glucose levels: these are usually very high
- U&Es, this usually shows high urea and creatinine levels, with a relatively larger impairment in urea (pre-renal renal failure)
- There is no acidosis in these patients (unless it is due to the precipitating cause)
- Investigations for causes of HONK are mandatory (CXR, ECG, urinalysis, CT head if necessary)
- Blood and urine cultures should be requested in all patients with HONK

Treatment of HONK
Treatment of HONK is broadly similar to that of DKA, but with some differences:
- Fluid
  - Fluid replacement should be more gentle in HONK compared with DKA as these are older patients, who are more prone to heart failure with aggressive fluid replacement. In difficult cases, a central line should be inserted to help guide the appropriate fluid replacement
- Potassium
  - In uncomplicated HONK, potassium levels do not drop particularly quickly due to the absence of acidosis, but this should still be carefully monitored
- Insulin
  - Despite the very high glucose levels in these patients, insulin requirements in HONK are modest and, therefore, insulin should be given at 0.5–2 units/h aiming for a gradual drop in blood sugar (around 5 mmol/L/h)
- Bicarbonate
  - This is not needed in uncomplicated hyperosmolar hyperglycaemia as the patient is not usually acidotic
- Precipitating cause(s)
  - Infection is the most common precipitating cause and, therefore, antibiotic cover must be started after appropriate cultures
- Other measures
  - Due to high osmolarity and dehydration, thrombotic complications are very common and, therefore, all patients should be covered with prophylactic unfractionated heparin
- Monitoring
  - This should be done regularly with blood samples taken every 2 h in the first 6–8 h to assess response to treatment

Hypoglycaemia
This is fully discussed in the neuroendocrine section of this book and, therefore, it will only be addressed here in relation to diabetes.
- Hypoglycaemia in diabetes patients may be secondary to oral hypoglycaemic agents (usually sulphonylurea) or insulin
- All patients with diabetes should be warned regarding hypoglycaemic symptoms:
  - Tremor and sweating
  - Nausea
  - Hunger
- Patients with hypoglycaemic symptoms should have their capillary glucose checked to confirm the diagnosis before initiating treatment
- Patients with frequent hypoglycaemic episodes may lose their warning symptoms, in which case plasma glucose should be kept slightly elevated for 2–3 weeks in order to regain the hypoglycaemic symptoms

Treatment of hypoglycaemia
- Patient conscious:
  - Oral glucose or sucrose (any fluid high in sugar content would do, such as Lucozade)
- Patient unconscious
  - Intravenous glucose
  - Intramuscular or s.c. glucagons (this loses its effect with repeated dosing)

Chronic complications
Investigations for chronic complications have been discussed above and only treatment is covered here.

Treatment of microvascular disease
- Retinopathy
  - Ensure good glucose control
  - Ensure good blood pressure control
  - Laser therapy in advanced stages
- Nephropathy
  - Early nephropathy (microalbuminuria): angiotensin converting enzyme inhibitors or angiotensin receptor blockers (sometimes a combination of the two) can be used to delay/prevent further deterioration in renal function. Also, need to ensure good glycaemia and blood pressure control
  - Advanced nephropathy (macroalbuminuria or raised creatinine): similar measures to those above can be used. Potassium and renal function should be frequently monitored and referral to a renal physician considered
  - End-stage renal disease: dialysis and renal transplant
- Neuropathy
  - Painless peripheral neuropathy: repeated foot examination by patient and/or cohabiting relative and regular chiropody
  - Charcot's arthopathy: immobilization of the joint is important to prevent further damage, and bisphosphonate may be of help
  - Painful peripheral neuropathy: difficult to treat and most only have a partial response. Some of the agents

used include: tricyclic antidepressants, capsaicin, anti-convulsants (phenytoin, gabapentin) and opiates

○ Autonomic neuropathy: postural drop in blood pressure can be treated with mechanical measures (wearing support stockings, sleeping with the head elevated) and fludrocortisone (monitor for hypertension and hypernatraemia). Gastrointestinal symptoms such as vomiting can be treated with metoclopramide, domperidone and erythromycin, and diarrhoea with loperamide

○ Sexual dysfunction: rule out an endocrine cause. Phosphodiesterase inhibitors, such as sildenafil, may help. Ensure good diabetes and blood pressure control

Treatment of macrovascular complications

- The majority of patients with diabetes die of cardio-vascular disease
- The risk of myocardial infarction in subjects with T2DM diabetes is similar to those without diabetes and a previous cardiac event
- Patients with diabetes and established cardiovascular disease are treated similarly to high risk non-diabetic individuals with known cardiovascular disease (discussed in the cardiovascular book of this series)
- Diabetes patients should, therefore, be treated with:
  ○ Lipid lowering agents such as statins (simvastatin, atorvastatin, rosuvastatin) to lower cholesterol levels and reduce cardiovascular events.
  ○ Other agents can also be used such as ezetimibe, which inhibits cholesterol absorption in the gut, and fibrates, which lower cholesterol levels but their main effect is on triglycerides
  ○ Angiotensin converting enzyme inhibitors (ACEI)
  ○ Antiplatelet agents (aspirin or clopidogrel)
  ○ Agents to maintain strict blood pressure control
  ○ Treat microalbuminuria, which is a cardiovascular risk

Lipid abnormalities and obesity

Lipid abnormalities

- The two main lipid molecules in the plasma are triglycerides and cholesterol
- To make these lipid particles water-soluble, they are bound to phospholipids and lipoproteins in plasma
- Lipid measurements are best performed on a fasting sample. The following measurements can be done:
  - Total cholesterol (TC) high levels are atherogenic. TC is composed of low-density lipoprotein cholesterol (LDLc) – high levels are associated with increased risk of vascular disease – and high-density lipoprotein cholesterol (HDLc) – low levels are associated with increased risk of vascular disease, whereas high levels are protective
  - Triglycerides: high levels are atherogenic and can also result in pancreatitis

Hyperlipidaemia

There are a number of different types of hyperlipidaemias, including:

- Isolated raised cholesterol
  - Polygenic hypercholesterolaemia: probably the commonest cause of isolated hypercholesterolaemia
  - Familial hypercholesterolaemia: an autosomal dominant condition affecting 1 : 500 people
- Isolated raised triglycerides
  - Autosomal dominant affecting around 1 : 300 people, characterized by eruptive xanthomas and pancreatitis
- Raised cholesterol and triglycerides
  - Familial combined hyperlipidaemia: occurs in 1 : 250 people
- Secondary causes of hyperlipidaemia
  - Diet excessive in fat

  - Diabetes mellitus: mainly affects triglyceride levels (increase) and HDL levels (decrease), particularly in those with poor glucose control
  - Hypothyroidism: affects LDL levels (increase)
  - Renal failure: affects LDL levels (increase), HDL (decrease) and triglycerides (increase)
  - Liver disease: obstructive liver lesions affect LDL levels (increase)
  - Drugs: a number of drugs can affect lipid levels including β-blockers, thiazide diuretics, steroids, protease inhibitors and alcohol

Clinical presentation

- Patients may be asymptomatic and hyperlipidaemia is picked up during routine testing
- Others can present with complications of hyperlipidaemia including:
  - Atherothrombotic disease (myocardial infarction, stroke)
  - Pancreatitis
- Individuals with secondary hyperlipidaemia present with symptoms of original disease

Treatment

- Lifestyle changes are important (diet, exercise and stopping smoking) as these simple measures can lower LDL and increased HDL levels
- For primary prevention (individuals with no previous complications due to hyperlipidaemia): there are special risk factor engines that calculate future cardiovascular risk and hyperlipidaemic agents are usually used in those with more than 20% risk over a 10-year period
- Individuals with a previous vascular event or high-risk subjects (for example diabetics), are treated with hyperlipidaemic agents even in the presence of normal lipid profile
- Agents used include statins, such as simvastatin, atorvastatin and rosuvastatin

Endocrinology and Diabetes: Clinical Cases Uncovered. By R. Ajjan. Published 2009 by Blackwell Publishing, ISBN: 978-1-4051-5726-1

○ Most widely used hyperlipidaemic agents due to their undoubted clinical benefits

○ Mode of action is related to decreased synthesis of cholesterol in the liver [inhibition of 3-hydroxy, 3-methylglutaryl coenzyme A (HMG CoA)]

○ Effective at reducing LDL levels, minor effect on HDL and triglycerides

○ Side effects are rare and include muscular aches and pains, derangement in liver function and rhabdomyolysis, a potentially life-threatening complication but fortunately very rare

All diabetes patients above the age of 40 are prescribed a statin (regardless of cholesterol levels), to reduce the risk of future vascular events

Ezetimibe

○ This agent reduces cholesterol absorption

○ Effective in combination with a statin but less impressive when used alone

• Fibrates

○ Effective at reducing triglycerides and, to a lesser extent, LDL levels. Also, they raise HDL levels

○ Their role in reducing cardiovascular risk is not as clear as statins

○ Usually used as second- or third-line treatment, except in those with isolated hypertriglyceridaemia, when fibrates are used as first-line treatment

• Nicotinic acid

○ Very effective at increasing HDL levels

○ The role of this agent in cardiovascular protection is unknown

○ Use is limited by side effects (severe flushing)

• Omega-3 fatty acids

○ Effective at reducing triglyceride levels

Obesity

• A major health problem in the developed world and it is on the increase

• Related largely to increased food intake and sedentary lifestyle

• Genetic factors play a role as some individuals are more susceptible to developing obesity

• There are some rare cases of obesity that have a clear genetic basis (monogenic obesity), including:

○ Leptin and leptin receptor deficiency

○ Prader-Willi syndrome

○ Laurence-Moon-Biedl syndrome

• Complications of obesity include:

○ Insulin resistance and diabetes mellitus

○ Lipid abnormalities

○ Cardiovascular disease

○ Hypertension

○ Mechanical joint pain and osteoarthritis

○ Sleep apnoea

○ Increased risk of cancers

○ Reproductive abnormalities (PCOS, impaired fertility)

Clinical presentation

• Concerns over body image secondary to obesity

• Complications (e.g. diabetes, cardiovascular disease)

Box 15 Obesity and BMI

• Obesity is assessed using body mass index (BMI), calculated by the formula: weight (kg)/[height(m)]^2

• BMI = 18.5–24.9: healthy

• BMI = 25–30: overweight

• BMI >30: obese

Investigations

• Fasting glucose (rule out diabetes)

• Fasting lipid profile

• Thyroid function tests

• ECG

• Specific tests in case of clinical suspicion (such as Cushing's syndrome for example)

Treatment

• Lifestyle changes

○ Diet: it is always useful to arrange an appointment with a dietician as minor changes in dietary habits can have a major influence on weight reduction

○ Increase exercise activity

• More severe dietary restrictions: those with severe obesity are sometimes admitted to hospital to initiate a very low calorie diet under clinical supervision

• Drug treatment

○ Orlistat inhibits gut lipase activity and reduces fat absorption. Patient should comply with low-fat diet. Side effects include diarrhoea (oily diarrhoea is characteristic), often in those who do not comply with reduction in fat intake

○ Sibutramine is a centrally acting appetite suppressant. Side effects include hypertension and increased heart rate, which limit its use

○ Rimonabant is a newer agent which acts on the cannabinoid receptor blocker resulting in reduced appetite, increased feeling of satiety, positive effect on plasma glucose and lipid profile and helps to quit smoking. Side effects include depression in up to 1 in 7 patients, individuals on antidepressants should not be prescribed this agent. Individuals should be observed closely for the development of this complication

- Surgery
  - Gastric bypass surgery is an effective treatment but reserved for those with severe obesity who are not responding to lifestyle changes and/or medical treatment

The neuroendocrine system

- Neuroendocrine cells are found in the gastrointestinal tract
- Benign and malignant tumours of the neuroendocrine system are rare and result in excess hormone production. Clinical manifestations differ according to the nature of the secreted hormone
- It should be noted that some of these tumours may also secrete pure endocrine hormones such as ACTH, PTH and GHRH resulting in Cushing's syndrome, hypercalcaemia and acromegaly respectively
- The characteristics of neuroendocrine tumours are summarized in Table 25

Insulinomas
- Insulinomas result in hypoglycaemia through excessive secretion of insulin
- These are usually benign and only around 10% show evidence of malignancy
- May be part of MEN-1 (see below)

Clinical presentation
- Symptoms of hypoglycaemia (usually relieved by eating)
  - Tremor and sweating
  - Nausea
  - Hunger
  - Weight gain secondary to frequent snacking (to avoid/treat hypoglycaemia)

Investigations
Fasting tests
- 16-h fast: the absence of hypoglycaemia after 16-h fast makes the diagnosis of insulinoma unlikely (test to be repeated three times)

Endocrinology and Diabetes: Clinical Cases Uncovered. By R. Ajjan. Published 2009 by Blackwell Publishing, ISBN: 978-1-4051-5726-1

- 72-h fast: this may be necessary in suspicious cases
  - Patient is admitted to hospital and fasted
  - Blood glucose and patient symptoms are regularly monitored
  - The presence of low glucose (<2.5 mmol/L) together with elevated insulin and C peptide confirms the diagnosis
  - It is important to measure C peptide to rule out exogenous administration of insulin (injected insulin has no C peptide, whereas endogenous insulin production is associated with detectable plasma levels of C peptide)

Localizing the tumour
- This can be difficult as tumours are often small
  - CT or MRI of the pancreas
  - Endoscopic ultrasound of the pancreas
  - Radiolabelled octreotide scanning: the majority of these tumours take up octreotide

Treatment
- Surgical removal is the treatment of choice
- Octreotide and/or diazoxide can be useful to reduce insulin secretion
- Malignant tumours with metastases: palliative treatment with streptozotocin or 5-fluorouracil

Carcinoid tumours
- The majority of these tumours develop in the gut but a minority can be found in the lungs and rarely other organs
- These tumours produce mainly serotonin (which is metabolized to 5-hydroxyindolacetic acid, 5HIAA)
- These tumours also have the ability to produce a large number of other hormones and proteins including ACTH, PTH, histamine and prostaglandin
- Carcinoid tumours are malignant but usually slow-growing and some patients live 20–30 years after the diagnosis

Table 25 Characteristics of the neuroendocrine tumours.

Excess hormone	Produced by	Clinical disease
Insulin	Pancreatic β-cells	Insulinoma
Serotonin, kinins	Intestine	Carcinoid syndrome
	Stomach	
	Pancreas	
Gastrin	Pancreatic G cells	Gastrinoma (Zollinger Ellison syndrome)
	Stomach	
	Small intestine	
Glucagon	Pancreatic α-cells	Glucagonoma
Somatostatin	Pancreatic δ-cells	Somatostatinoma
	Stomach	
	Small intestine	
Vasoactive intestinal peptide (VIP)	Pancreatic VIP cells	VIPoma

Clinical presentation

- Flushing, can be precipitated by:
  - Alcohol
  - Spicy food
  - Exercise
  - Carcinoid flush usually affects the face and upper thorax and is shown in Fig. 38 (colour plate section)
- Diarrhoea
- Asthma
- Right valvular heart lesions: fibrosis of right heart valves, which may be due to serotonin
- Pellagra-like skin lesions (excessive tryptophan metabolism results in nicotinamide deficiency)

It should be noted that individuals with carcinoid syndrome due to gastrointestinal tumours will only be symptomatic if they have liver metastases, in contrast to bronchial carcinoid subjects, who develop the symptoms before metastases have taken place.

Investigations

- Urinary 5-HIAA levels are elevated in the majority of patients and have a high specificity
- Plasma chromogranin A: higher sensitivity than 5-HIAA but lower specificity
- Imaging
  - CT/MRI of chest and/or abdomen
  - Octreotide scanning

Treatment

- Surgical removal
- Somatostatin analogues for residual disease or if surgery is contraindicated
- Palliative therapy
  - Hepatic embolization: using angiography techniques
  - Chemotherapy: streptozotocin and 5-fluorouracil
  - Immunotherapy: α-interferon: useful in controlling symptoms and can be combined with octreotide

Gastrinomas

- Two-thirds of these tumours are malignant
- Excessive gastrin secretion results in increased acid secretion by the stomach

Clinical presentation

- Recurrent peptic ulcer disease that is refractory to treatment
- Malabsorption and diarrhoea

Investigations

- Inappropriately elevated gastrin levels in the presence of increased stomach acid secretion confirms the diagnosis
- Imaging
  - As described under insulinoma

Treatment

- Surgical removal is the treatment of choice
- Proton pump inhibitors (omeprazole, lansoprazole) for those with residual tumour or in whom surgery is contraindicated

Glucagonomas

- Two-thirds of these tumours are malignant but they are slow-growing

Clinical presentation

- Skin rash: necrolytic migratory erythema, can precede the diagnosis by many years
- Glucose intolerance and diabetes: due to excess glucagon secretion
- Mucous membrane involvement: stomatitis and glossitis

Investigations

- Raised plasma glucagon in the presence of symptoms/signs is diagnostic

- Localization
  - CT or MRI of the abdomen
  - Octreotide scanning: particularly useful to evaluate the extent of metastases

Treatment

- Surgery: cure rate is unfortunately very low (<10%)
- Octreotide or long acting somatostatin analogues can be very useful to control symptoms
- Palliative treatment with streptozotocin or 5-fluorouacil

Somatostatinomas

- These are very rare with an incidence of 1 in 40 million
- Characterized by:
  - Glucose intolerance and diabetes mellitus
  - Gall stones
  - Diarrhoea and malabsorption

VIPoma

- Very rare and characterized by:
  - Watery diarrhoea
  - Hypokalaemia

Neuroendocrine syndromes

These describe the association of a number of neuroendocrine abnormalities and include:

- Multiple endocrine neoplasia type 1
  - An autosomal dominant condition (gene on chromosome 11, *menin* gene is affected), with a prevalence of 1 in 10000
  - Tumours occur in two or more endocrine glands: parathyroid (hyperplasia or adenoma), almost all cases; pancreas (insulinoma, gastrinoma), 70% of patients; pituitary (prolactinoma, acromegaly), 30% of patients. The easiest way to remember this is PPP (parathyroid, pancreas, pituitary)
- Multiple endocrine neoplasia type 2
  - An autosomal dominant condition (gene of chromosome 10, *ret* protooncogene is affected)
  - Around one-third of gene carriers do not manifest clinically significant disease
  - Tumours occur in two or more endocrine glands: thyroid gland (medullary thyroid cancer), often the presenting feature; adrenal glands (pheochromocytomas), in 50% of patients; parathyroid glands, in 30% of patients. The way to remember this is TAP (thyroid, adrenal, parathyroid)

Table 26 Summary of the clinical presentation of different neuroendocrine tumours.

Neuroendocrine tumour	Clinical presentation
Insulinoma	Symptoms of hypoglycaemia
	Weight gain
Carcinoid syndrome	Flushing
	Diarrhoea
	Asthma
	Right-sided heart lesions
	Pellagra-like skin lesions
Gastrinoma (Zollinger Ellison syndrome)	Recurrent and refractory peptic ulcer disease
Glucagonoma	Typical skin rash (necrolytic migratory erythema)
	Glucose intolerance
Somatostatinoma	Glucose intolerance
	Gall stones
	Diarrhoea and malabsorption
VIPoma	Watery diarrhoea

Some patients may have mucosal neuromas and a marfanoid habitus and these are classified as MEN 2B.

- Von Hippel-Lindau disease
  - An autosomal dominant condition
  - Clinical manifestations include: pheochromocytoma, bilateral in half the patients; pancreatic neuroendocrine tumours; retinal and central nervous system hemangiomas; and renal cell carcinoma (the usual cause of death in these patients)
- Neurofibromatosis (NF)
  - NF1 is an autosomal dominant condition characterized by: multiple neurofibromas, café-au-lait spots, iris lisch nodule, pheochromocytoma and gut endocrine tumours
  - NF1 should be differentiated from NF2, which is characterized by: disorders of the central nervous system (meningiomas), cranial nerve tumours (usually optic glioma); NF2 is not associated with endocrine abnormalities

The main clinical characteristics of the neuroendocrine tumours are summarized in Table 26.

Case 1 A 19-year-old with abdominal pain and vomiting

Kathryn, a 19-year-old student, who is usually fit and well, is admitted to accident and emergency (A&E) with a 2-day history of abdominal pain, vomiting and feeling generally unwell. She has lost 5 kg in weight over the past 3 weeks for no clear reason. There is no significant past medical history of note except for three episodes of urinary tract infection (UTI) over the past 6 months.

What are the differential diagnoses of abdominal pain and vomiting?
Intra-abdominal pathology
- Peptic ulcer disease
- Pancreatitis
- Cholecystitis and gall stones
- Appendicitis
- Ectopic pregnancy
- Intestinal obstruction
- Renal calculi and pyelonephritis

Other conditions associated with abdominal pain but less likely to cause vomiting
- Dysmenorrhea
- Pelvic inflammatory disease
- Inflammatory bowel disease
- Intra-abdominal arterial and venous thrombosis
- Ruptured aortic aneurysm (in older individuals)

Endocrine causes of abdominal pain and vomiting
- Diabetes mellitus complicated by diabetic ketoacidosis
- Hypoadrenalism
- Hypercalcaemia

Endocrinology and Diabetes: Clinical Cases Uncovered. By R. Ajjan.
Published 2009 by Blackwell Publishing, ISBN: 978-1-4051-5726-1

What clinical features are associated with weight loss?
- Chronic infections and infestations: particularly in individuals with a deranged immune system, such as patients with AIDS
- Malignancy
- Diabetes mellitus
- Hyperthyroidism
- Malnutrition: uncommon in Western countries
- Degenerative neurological and muscular diseases

It is impossible to give an accurate diagnosis at this stage and a more detailed history and careful physical examination is of paramount importance in order to establish the correct diagnosis.

What questions will you ask?
- Has the pain and vomiting started recently or has it been occurring for weeks, months or years?
- Was the onset of pain sudden or gradual?
- What is the pain like and how severe is it?
- Where is the pain localized?
- Does anything relieve the pain?
- Has a new treatment been introduced recently?
- Are there any associated symptoms (review of systems)?

On further questioning, Kathryn tells you that the abdominal pain was gradual in onset over 4–6 h, generalized and cramp-like, with severity varying between 2/10 and 4/10. Nausea and vomiting preceded the abdominal pain by 6 h or so. Kathryn has been on oral contraceptive pills (OCP) for 18 months and her last withdrawal bleed was 1 week ago.

Does this help with the diagnosis?
- The gradual onset of pain and low severity (although this is subjective) make a surgical cause for the pain less likely, but do not fully rule it out. For example, appendi-

citis may initially present with gradual and cramp-like abdominal pain. Also, it should be noted that in some cases of acute abdomen, the symptoms may be relatively mild and this can be seen in older patients or in individuals who are on steroid treatment

• The combination of OCP use and a recent normal withdrawal bleeding rules out dysmenorrhea and ectopic pregnancy as causes for Kathryn's pain

During review of systems and on further questioning, Kathryn tells you that she had polyuria up to 15 times/day and nocturia 6 times/night for 2 weeks prior to her current presentation. She is a non-smoker and drinks up to 20 units of alcohol per week. Family history includes pernicious anaemia in her uncle and hypothyroidism in her mother.

Does this help with the diagnosis?

Polyuria can be secondary to a number of causes. In this case, a urinary tract infection may have caused the abdominal pain and polyuria, which is usually associated with dysuria, and only small amounts of urine are passed on each occasion.

Box 16 Other causes of polyuria

• Electrolyte abnormalities such as hypercalcaemia
• Chronic renal disease
• Endocrine disease such as diabetes insipidus (lack of, or ineffective, antidiuretic hormone)
• Osmotic diuresis due to high plasma glucose levels (diabetes mellitus)
• The use of drugs such as lithium and demeclocycline

In this patient:
• Hypercalcaemia can indeed cause abdominal pain and polyuria but this condition is infrequently seen in a young person. Nevertheless, it should be checked out
• There is no indication that this patient has chronic renal disease but this should certainly be excluded. The fact that she had three UTIs in 6 months may indicate a pathology in the urinary tract. However, urinary infections are common in female individuals, particularly if they are sexually active
• Diabetes insipidus is a recognized cause of polyuria but is not associated with abdominal pain or vomiting and therefore this diagnosis is unlikely
• Type 1 diabetes mellitus (T1DM) is a strong possibility. Diabetic ketoacidosis (DKA), a complication of T1DM, classically presents with:

◦ Nausea
◦ Vomiting
◦ Abdominal pain
◦ Associated symptoms: a few days/weeks history of polyuria and polydipsia (known as osmotic symptoms), and weight loss

The family history of autoimmunity further supports this diagnosis, as it suggests a genetic predisposition to autoimmune disease in Kathryn

Kathryn deteriorates and becomes slightly confused, with a drop in her Glasgow Coma Scale (GCS) from 15/15 to 13/15 (E3, V5, M5). On examination, she is tired, dehydrated, tachycardic at 112 beats/min, has a temperature of 36.6°C, blood pressure of 115/70 mmHg, with a postural drop of 20/10 mmHg, and respiratory rate of 32/min, with otherwise normal chest examination. Cardiac auscultation is normal, and abdominal palpation reveals minimal generalized tenderness with no rigidity, guarding or rebound tenderness.

How do her clinical findings help with the diagnosis?

• Kathryn is clinically dehydrated with tachycardia and a postural drop in blood pressure indicating significant fluid loss
• The tachypnea is a matter of concern and could be due to a primary lung pathology or secondary causes. A primary lung pathology in this patient may be:

◦ Chest infection may result in tachypnea and pneumonia is a recognized cause of abdominal pain. However, she is apyrexial and chest auscultation is unremarkable, making this an unlikely diagnosis
◦ Pulmonary embolus causes tachypnea and hypotension, and OCP use is a known risk factor for thromboembolism. However, Kathyrn has no chest pain, whereas abdominal pain and vomiting are not usually features of pulmonary embolism
◦ Metabolic acidosis: the respiratory system compensates for metabolic acidosis by increasing the respiratory rate to blow off CO_2, resulting in respiratory alkalosis, which may fully or partially compensate for the metabolic acidosis. Causes of metabolic acidosis are summarized in Table 27 and DKA is one cause, which seems to fit the diagnosis. A distinctive ketotic-smelling breath can further aid the diagnosis of DKA.

• Abdominal examination revealed only minimal generalized tenderness with no signs of acute abdomen (rigidity, guarding or rebound tenderness), which is reassuring

Table 27 Causes of metabolic acidosis.

Metabolic acidosis with increased anion gap (increased acid production/ingestion)	Metabolic acidosis with normal anion gap (imbalance between HCO_3^- and H^+ ions)
Lactic acidosis: increased production of lactate due to infection, shock or hypoxia	Renal tubular acidosis: loss of HCO_3^- or excessive absorption of H^+ ions
Uraemic acidosis: renal failure	Diarrhoea: loss of HCO_3^-
Ketotic acidosis: diabetes or alcohol	Pancreatic fistula: loss of HCO_3^-
Toxins and drugs: salicylate overdose, ethylene glycol and methanol ingestion	Addison's disease: excessive absorption of H^+ ions
	Drugs: acetozolamide: excessive absorption of H^+ ions

and makes a surgical cause for Kathryn's abdominal pain less likely

What test(s) would you request to confirm the diagnosis?

Taken together, the most likely diagnosis here is DKA, which is characterized by:
• Metabolic acidosis
• Raised plasma glucose
• Dehydration
• Increased ketone production

Therefore, the following tests should be requested:
• Venous bicarbonate and pH: bicarbonate falls in DKA to <15 mmol/L and can be as low as 1 mmol/L, resulting in a variable degree of acidosis. In early DKA, pH can be normal due to compensated respiratory alkalosis. A common hospital practice is to take an arterial blood sample for bicarbonate and pH measurement (arterial blood gas analysis), which is unnecessary unless a primary lung pathology precipitating DKA is suspected
• Plasma glucose: this is elevated in DKA. Capillary glucose (finger-prick glucose) can be initially done to give a quick result but it should always be followed by plasma glucose measurement
• U&Es: in DKA these show:
  ○ High or high-normal urea (due to dehydration)
  ○ High or high-normal potassium (due to acidosis)
  ○ In advanced or more severe cases, creatinine can be elevated (due to pre-renal renal failure)
• Urine dipstick: detection of large amounts of ketone bodies in the urine aids the diagnosis of DKA

In addition to DKA-specific tests, other blood tests should be requested, including:
• Full blood count: usually requested in ill individuals

attending A&E, and can aid in the diagnosis of anaemia (low haemoglobin) and infection (raised white cells). It is worth bearing in mind that infection may precipitate DKA
• Cultures: DKA can be precipitated by an infection and, therefore, blood and urine cultures (as well as culture of sputum if respiratory symptoms are present) are usually requested on presentation, unless the cause of DKA is clear (non-compliance with insulin injections for example)
• Chest X-ray: to rule chest infection as the precipitating cause. This is perhaps not necessary in newly diagnosed patients with no reason to suspect a respiratory pathology
• Electrocardiogram: this should be requested in patients with diabetes particularly in the older age group as silent myocardial infarction (myocardial infarction with no chest pain) is common in these patients and may precipitate DKA. A myocardial infarction is unlikely here due to Kathryn's young age but an ECG may show abnormalities and arrhythmias consistent with electrolyte disturbances (hyperkalaemia for example), which may require urgent attention
• Abdominal X-ray (AXR): this is usually requested in patients attending A&E with severe abdominal pain and vomiting to rule out intestinal obstruction and/or perforation. Opinions will differ, but an AXR is probably not necessary here as Kathryn has no signs to suggest an acute abdomen

Blood, urine and radiological tests show the following:
FBC: Hb 14.1 g/L
*   WBC 23.3× 10⁹/L (neutrophils 18.2× 10⁹/L)*
*   Platelets 380 × 10⁹/L*

U&Es: Na 131 mmol/L

          K 5.4 mmol/L

          Urea 10.1 mmol/L

          Creatinine 124 µmol/L

          Bicarbonate 9 mmol/L

          pH 7.16

Glucose   22 mmol/L

Amylase   normal

CXR   clear

AXR   normal

Urine dipstick: ketones +++, glucose +++, RBC –, WBC –,
   nitrates –

Box 17 Precipitants of DKA

- New diagnosis of T1DM in 20% of cases
- In a known diabetic patient, DKA can be due to:
  ○ Infection in 35% cases
  ○ Non-compliance with insulin injection in 30%
  ○ Errors in insulin administration and dose calculation in 15%
  ○ In a minority of patients, DKA may be precipitated by an ischaemic event such as myocardial infarction

---

How do you interpret these results?

- Kathryn has high WBC with elevated neutrophil counts suggesting an underlying infection. However, DKA patients may have very high WBC count without associated infection, which normalizes once DKA is adequately treated. In some cases, infection is difficult to rule out, and this is why a septic screen is requested (blood and urine cultures, sputum culture if any, CXR), followed by antibiotic cover if the suspicion of infection is high
- The diagnosis of metabolic acidosis is evident from the combination of low pH and low bicarbonate
- The metabolic acidosis together with high plasma glucose and strongly positive urinary ketones confirm the diagnosis of DKA
  ○ Patients with DKA excrete large amounts of ketones in their urine due to deranged glucose metabolism and the production of abnormally high levels of ketone bodies: acetone, acetoacetate, β-hydroxybutarate
  ○ Urine dip testing methods check only for acetone and acetoacetate
- Other abnormalities include:
  ○ High urea consistent with dehydration
  ○ High potassium secondary to acidosis, which shifts the potassium from the intracellular compartment to the extracellular space. Potassium falls with successful treatment of DKA and this should be monitored carefully as detailed below
  ○ Marginally low sodium is commonly seen in patients with DKA due to high plasma glucose and this normalizes with treatment of the condition and the fall in blood sugar
- Urine dipstick is positive for ketones and glucose consistent with the diagnosis of DKA. Of note is the absence of pyuria and nitrates on urine dipstick, making the diagnosis of a urinary tract infection unlikely

How would you manage this patient?

The management should be directed to:
- Correct the metabolic abnormality by replacing:
  ○ Fluid
  ○ Insulin
  ○ Potassium
- Treat the precipitating cause (if any)
- Monitor the patient carefully during treatment of DKA

Local hospital guidelines should be followed for the management of patients with DKA

Fluid

- Fluid replacement usually starts with normal saline (0.9%): 1 L over the first h, 1 L over 2 h then 1 L every 4–6 h, with careful monitoring of the patient clinical status and urine output
- Fluid replacement should be modified according to the clinical status of the patient. For example, if the patient has a very low blood pressure at presentation with signs of shock, initial fluid replacement should be more aggressive
- Normal saline should continue until the blood glucose drops below 12–15 mmol/L (different protocols use different cut-offs), when saline should be substituted with 5% glucose. This helps to restore normal energy metabolism and clears the blood of ketone bodies, thereby normalizing the pH

Potassium

- Monitoring of potassium status is very important as failure to replace potassium can result in severe hypokalaemia, which may cause cardiac arrhythmias, potentially resulting in death
- Serum potassium is usually elevated on initial presentation due to the presence of acidosis, but it quickly drops after the initiation of treatment (both insulin replace-

Table 28 An example of sliding scale insulin. This is only a guide and different sliding scales can be used as some individuals require higher doses of insulin whereas others need less.

Capillary glucose	Insulin dose
<4.0 mmol/L	0.5 units/h (with i.v. dextrose): review
4.1–10.0 mmol/L	2 unit/h
10.0–16.0 mmol/L	4 units/h
>16.0 mmol/L	6 units/h: review

ment and correction of acidosis shift the potassium from the extracellular space into the cells)
• As a rough guide:
  ○ 20 mmol/L potassium should be added to i.v. fluid in patients with normokalaemia
  ○ 40 mmol/L to those with hypokalaemia
  ○ No potassium should be given to those with hyperkalaemia

Insulin
• Insulin is started as an i.v. infusion at around 0.1 U/kg/h and adjusted according to a sliding scale insulin (see Table 28)
• Some diabetologists feel that a sliding scale insulin should be avoided in DKA patients (to avoid too many insulin dose adjustments) and the insulin dose should be regularly reviewed and adjusted by an experienced doctor. However, this can be difficult practically and, therefore, a simple sliding scale is used in most hospitals
• A common practice is to give a starting dose of 4–6 units of insulin/h and modify the dose according to plasma glucose levels
• Intravenous insulin should only be stopped when the urine is ketone-free and the patient is clinically well

Bicarbonate
• This is very rarely given; only in cases of severe acidosis not responding to conventional treatment
• Bicarbonate administration should only be done in an intensive care setting and after the involvement of senior clinicians with expertise in DKA management

Precipitating cause(s)
• Around two-thirds of DKA cases are due to newly diagnosed type 1 diabetes or compliance problems/errors in insulin administration in known diabetic patients

• In around one-third, DKA is due to other causes such as infection or myocardial infarction and these conditions should be treated appropriately

Other measures
• Low-dose heparin to prevent thromboembolism is recommended by some, but there is no clear evidence to support this practice, which is unnecessary unless other risk factors exist (prolonged immobility)
• A nasogastric tube should be inserted into patients with protracted vomiting

Monitoring
• Capillary glucose should be checked hourly
• Potassium levels should be regularly assessed and this can be done using the following time points as a guide: presentation (time 0 h), 2 h, 4 h, 8 h, 16 h and 24 h
• Both venous bicarbonate and glucose can also be checked at the same time points as above to assess response to treatment
• The above time points can be modified according to the severity of the DKA and the response to treatment
   The management of DKA is summarized in Fig. 37 (Part 1, p. 57).

What is the prognosis in this case?
Prognosis is very good in uncomplicated DKA and the mortality rate is less than 3%.

Kathryn improves after initial treatment, her BP normalizes and her confusion clears. However, she starts feeling very weak 12 h after admission and complains of palpitations. An ECG is shown (Fig. 39).

What complication has occurred? How should this be treated?
• ECG shows changes consistent with hypokalaemia
  ○ ST depression
  ○ Presence of U wave after T wave
• Plasma potassium should be checked and corrected *urgently*:
  ○ Supplementation of potassium to i.v. fluid
  ○ A cardiac monitor should be attached to the patient

Twenty hours after admission, Kathryn's blood glucose levels fall to 6.8 mmol/L and the acidosis clears. However, Kathryn becomes suddenly confused and agitated and subsequently GCS drops to 6.

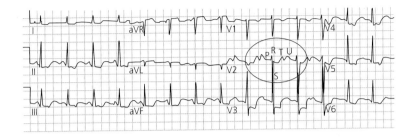

Figure 39

What urgent test would you request at this stage?

- A drop of GCS and neurological signs in a treated DKA patient should raise the suspicion of cerebral oedema, which may be secondary to over-enthusiastic fluid replacement
- This complication is rarely seen in adults but it is not uncommon in children
- If cerebral oedema is suspected, urgent CT/MRI of the head should be requested, and if the diagnosis is confirmed:
  - The patient should be immediately transferred to an intensive care unit
  - Should be treated with mannitol and dexamethasone, which may help to reduce the cerebral oedema
  - Unfortunately, prognosis is poor once this complication occurs, with mortality approaching 90% in adults

What does long-term management of a type 1 diabetes patient involve?

- Ensure strict glucose control
  - Monitored by home sugar readings and glycosylated haemoglobin levels (HbA1c). The input of the diabetes nurse specialist is important to provide support to patients and help with adjustments of insulin doses
  - Most commonly used insulin injection regimes in type 1 diabetes include four daily injections (one long acting and three short acting insulin with meals) or two daily injections with a mixture of short and long acting insulin preparations. An insulin pump can be used for those with erratic glucose control
  - Good diabetes control is important to avoid long-term microvascular complications (retinopathy, nephropathy and neuropathy) as well as macrovascular complications (coronary artery disease, cerebrovascular and peripheral vascular disease)
  - Tight glucose control should not be achieved at the expense of increasing hypoglycaemia, which can be dangerous and sometimes fatal
- Screen for the development of microvascular complications
  - Yearly retinal screening
  - Yearly check of urinary microalbumin: usually done on an early morning urine sample with results expressed as albumin/creatinine ratio (ACR)
  - Yearly foot examination to rule out neuropathy: usually done using monofilament test
- Watch for/prevent the development of macrovascular complications
  - Have a role threshold for investigating individuals with suspected vascular pathology
  - Add statin treatment to patients above the age of 40 or earlier in those at high risk
  - Adding aspirin treatment to high-risk individuals is of debatable benefit
  - Aggressively treat hypertension

CASE REVIEW

Kathryn is a young woman admitted to hospital with short history of abdominal pain, vomiting and feeling unwell. Also, there is a history of significant weight loss over a 3-week period. The differential diagnosis of abdominal pain is wide and a detailed history together with a full examination usually help to rule out a surgical cause, which should be diagnosed early as delays can have serious consequences. There is nothing in the history or examination to suggest an acute abdomen, and, therefore, a surgical cause for this patient's symptoms is less likely.

Continued

Kathryn's clinical condition subsequently deteriorates and her Glasgow Coma Scale (GCS) drops from 15/15 to 13/15. She is found to be clinically dehydrated, tachycardic and tachypneic. Taken together, diabetic ketoacidosis is suspected, which is subsequently confirmed by demonstrating low plasma pH and bicarbonate levels, raised glucose and significant ketonuria. Appropriate tests are arranged to rule out an underlying infection (CXR, blood cultures) and she is treated with intravenous fluid and insulin with initial improvement in her symptoms. However, 12 h after her admission, she starts complaining of palpitations; an ECG shows an abnormal U wave and a depressed ST segment. This was due to hypokalaemia

and inadequate monitoring of her potassium levels, which can fall very rapidly during DKA treatment. She is treated with intravenous fluid containing potassium, which stabilizes her condition, but she deteriorates again 24 h after admission and her GCS drops to 6. This raises the possibility of cerebral oedema and an urgent CT or MRI of the head should be requested. If confirmed this complication should be aggressively treated in intensive care settings.

DKA is a common condition and frequently the first presentation of diabetes. Monitoring is a vital part in the management, in order to avoid the development of serious complications, which may have tragic consequences.

KEY POINTS

- Diabetic ketoacidosis (DKA) is a relatively common condition, which can be life-threatening
- Abdominal pain, vomiting and tachypnea (air hunger) are typical manifestations of this diabetic complication
- DKA should be suspected in any type 1 diabetes patient with gastrointestinal symptoms. In those with no history of diabetes, DKA should be suspected in individuals, particularly the young, who are acutely unwell and have the above symptoms
- Around one-third of patients with DKA present as a new diagnosis of diabetes, one-third are due to errors or non-compliance with insulin administration in a known diabetes patient, and in the final third the DKA arises secondary to infections or an ischaemic event
- A history of osmotic symptoms, with or without weight loss, should prompt appropriate investigations to rule out diabetes as a cause
- Biochemical abnormalities in DKA include:
  - ○ Raised blood glucose
  - ○ Low bicarbonate with or without low pH
  - ○ Low pCO_2 on arterial blood gas analysis (not necessary to make the diagnosis)
  - ○ Heavy ketonuria

- Treatments for DKA include:
  - ○ Intravenous fluid (with adequate potassium replacement)
  - ○ Intravenous insulin
  - ○ Treat the precipitating cause
  - ○ Monitoring of glucose, bicarbonate and potassium is paramount to assess response to treatment
  - ○ Intravenous fluid and insulin should be continued until bicarbonate normalizes and the urine is ketone-free
- Serious complications of DKA include:
  - ○ Hypokalaemia (common)
  - ○ Cerebral oedema (rare)
- Long-term management of type 1 diabetes patients should include:
  - ○ Good glucose control
  - ○ Screen for the development of complications: for microvascular disease use retinal screening, urinary microalbumin and regular foot examination; for macrovascular disease, promptly investigate potential vascular pathology, initiate statin treatment for individuals at high risk or those above the age of 40 and aggressively treat hypertension and microalbuminuria

Case 2 A 35-year-old woman with palpitation and irritability

Andrea is a 35-year-old solicitor who presents with a 10-day history of constant palpitations, weakness and irritability.

What is the differential diagnosis and how would you proceed?

Palpitation is a common complaint and is a perception of 'increased' heart action. It can be physiological or pathological:

- Physiological: stressful life events can result in palpitation. A classical example is palpitations experienced by university students or junior doctors sitting an important exam
- Pathological: cardiac tachyarrhythmias (fast regular or irregular heart rate) may be due to:
  - A primary heart problem: in young patients, tachyarrhythmias, such as supraventricular tachycardia, commonly occur with no significant structural cardiac abnormality but may sometimes be secondary to serious cardiac abnormalities. However, these are usually intermittent and do not persist for 10 days as in this case
  - Non-cardiac palpitations: the commonest cause is hyperthyroidism and, therefore, it is important to rule this out in our patient

A detailed history and examination is required at this stage.

On further questioning Andrea tells you that she has had a number of symptoms for the past week, including: heat intolerance, hand tremor, generalized weakness, inability to sleep and frequent bowel motions. Her past medical history includes eczema localized to her hands, which is longstanding. Family history includes ischaemic heart disease in her father, diagnosed after a myocardial infarction at the age of 72, her mother suffers from vitiligo and her sister has type 1 diabetes.

Endocrinology and Diabetes: Clinical Cases Uncovered. By R. Ajjan. Published 2009 by Blackwell Publishing, ISBN: 978-1-4051-5726-1

How would this information help you in the diagnosis?

- Heat intolerance, hand tremor, loose bowel motions and weakness are all classical features of hyperthyroidism (symptoms of hyperthyroidism are summarized in Table 8, p. 16), making this diagnosis a real possibility
- There is a personal history of atopy and a family history of autoimmune diseases, suggesting a genetic predisposition to autoimmunity in Andrea
- The family history of ischaemic heart disease is probably irrelevant as it did not occur at a young age and myocardial infarction is not uncommon in men above the age of 70

How would you proceed here?

Having taken the history, physical examination is the next step, with special emphasis on the assessment of thyroid status. The signs of hyperthyroidism are summarized in Table 8, p. 16.

On examination, Andrea has sweaty palms with a marked hand tremor. Her pulse is regular at 104 beats/min and her BP is 110/70 with no postural drop. She has a marked lid lag.

How would you interpret these findings, and what other examination(s) would you do and why?

Andrea has clinical hyperthyroidism supported by the presence of: hand tremor, sweaty palms, tachycardia and lid lag. The next step would be directed at establishing the aetiology. Hyperthyroidism is due to Graves' disease (GD) in 80% of cases, and, therefore, it is important to look for specific signs of GD, including:

- Smooth symmetrical thyroid goitre
- Graves' ophthalmopathy (GO)
- Pretibial myxoedema

Andrea has eye signs similar to the patient shown in Fig. 40 (colour plate section). What abnormality do you see? How would that help in the diagnosis?

- The patient has proptosis, marked periorbital oedema and conjunctival injection, indicating the presence Graves' ophthalmopathy
- This is pathognomic for GD and is clinically evident in around 50% of patients with the disease

How would you clinically assess the severity of the eye condition? What associated condition would you look for?

The following signs are indications for urgent ophthalmology review:

- Failure of full eye closure
- Significant ophthalmoplegia
- Evidence of optic nerve compression

The presence of a skin condition called pretibial myxoedema in a patient with hyperthyroidism is also diagnostic of GD but this is found in less than 10% of GD patients and is almost always associated with clinically detectable GO.

What would you like to do next?

A neck examination; this usually reveals a smooth and symmetrical goitre in patients with GD.

What blood tests would you request?

This patient should have her thyroid function (TFTs) checked.

Her TFTs show the following (normal ranges):

- Free T4 24.2 pmol/L (10.0–25.0)
- TSH <0.05 mIU/L (0.2–6.0)

How do you interpret these results? What would you do?

- This patient has a normal FT4, suggesting euthyroidism
- TSH is suppressed, consistent with hyperthyroidism
- The most likely explanation for these results is T3 toxicosis, where the thyroid produces excess T3 without significant increase in T4 production
- Therefore, T3 levels should be requested

Her free T3 is 17.5 pmol/L (normal range 3.4–7.2).

What conclusion would you make?

This patient has hyperthyroidism due to T3 toxicosis secondary to GD

What other tests can be requested in patients with hyperthyroidism?

- Thyroid peroxidase antibodies are positive in up to 80% of GD patients
- Thyroid stimulating hormone receptor (TSHR) antibodies are positive in around 99% of patients if sensitive methods are used. However, these are not routinely requested and are reserved for difficult cases and for pregnant patients

What is the treatment of Graves' disease?

There are three treatment options for patients with Graves' disease: medical treatment, radioactive iodine and surgery.

Medical treatment

This is used to:

- Control thyroid function
- Induce remission

The most commonly used antithyroid drugs are carbimazole and propylthiouracil. These can be given as:

- A 'block and replace regime': a high dose of the drug is used and once the hyperthyroidism is brought under control, L-thyroxine (T4) is added to avoid hypothyroidism
- Titration regime: once euthyroidism is achieved by high-dose antithyroid drug, a low maintenance dose is given to keep the patient euthyroid

In the block and replace regime, treatment continues for 6–12 months, whereas 18 months is usually required using the titration regime. Once the treatment is stopped, the chances of disease remission are around 50%.

> **!RED FLAG**
>
> An important side effect, albeit rare, of antithyroid drugs is agranulocytosis and all patients are advised to seek IMMEDIATE medical attention if they develop a sore throat, mouth ulcers or high temperature to rule out this serious, and potentially, fatal complication of treatment.

Radioactive iodine (RAI)

This is administered orally, usually as a capsule, and it controls hyperthyroidism in the majority of patients. A minority of patients need a second, and rarely a third, dose. A large proportion of patients become hypothyroid with radioactive iodine therapy and will, therefore, require thyroxine replacement therapy for life. RAI is contraindicated in:

- Children
- Pregnant and lactating women
- Patients with urinary incontinence
- Patients who cannot comply with the safety precautions following RAI treatment
- This treatment is best avoided in patients with moderate to severe active GO, particularly smokers, as RAI may worsen the eye condition. In patients with active eye signs in whom RAI treatment cannot be avoided, it is advisable to cover with steroids starting just before RAI treatment and continuing with a reducing dosing regime for around 6 weeks

Surgery

This is reserved for the following patients:

- Failed or contraindicated medical therapy
- Unwilling to have RAI or in whom it is contraindicated
- Graves' disease and a suspicious thyroid nodule
- Graves' disease and compressive symptoms
- Patient preference
  Early complications of thyroid surgery include:
- Recurrent laryngeal nerve damage
- Hypocalcaemia
- Local haemorrhage
- Wound infection
- Thyroid storm in patients who are poorly prepared for surgery
  Late complications include:
- Hoarse voice (secondary to recurrent laryngeal nerve damage)
- Hypothyroidism
- Hypocalcaemia

Three months later, Andrea brings her friend to see you, who has had classical symptoms of hyperthyroidism, including hand tremor, increased sweating and palpitations, for a week. All these symptoms started following a flu-like illness. On examination, she has signs suggestive of hyperthyroidism, including a marked tremor and tachycardia, but she has no eye signs or skin abnormality. No goitre is seen on neck inspection; neck palpation is difficult due to exquisite tenderness in the area of the thyroid gland but no clear goitre is palpated.

Her TFTs show:
FT4 39 pmol/L
TSH <0.05 mIU/L
TSHR-antibodies negative
Andrea is concerned about the possibility of thyrotoxicosis due to Graves' disease.

Do you agree with her? Why? What other blood test would you request?

This patient is unlikely to have Graves' disease, because:

- She has pain and severe tenderness in her neck, which are not usual features of Graves' disease
- She does not seem to have a goitre
- She has no eye signs to suggest Graves' ophthalmopathy, nor does she have pretibial myxoedema
- Her symptoms followed a recent viral/bacterial infection
- Her TSHR antibodies are negative (see p. 15)

  Taken together (recent infection, thyrotoxicosis, severe neck tenderness), the likely diagnosis is De Quervain's thyroiditis, which usually occurs after upper respiratory infections, and thyrotoxicosis is due to thyroid destruction with consequent release of thyroid hormones, and not thyroid hormone overproduction by thyroid cells. In thyroiditis, inflammatory markers are raised and, therefore, C-reactive protein (CRP) should be requested.

What test would you request to *confirm* the diagnosis?

Thyroid uptake scan would confirm the diagnosis. In Graves' disease there is a uniform increased uptake in the thyroid gland due to over-activity of the thyroid cells, whereas in thyroiditis there is absent uptake due to thyroid destruction, as shown in Fig. 41.

How would you treat this patient?

Treatment is supportive:

- β-blockers can be given to control the symptoms of thyrotoxicosis
- Pain killers and non-steroidal anti-inflammatory agents are given to control the pain
- Rarely, in severe cases, short courses of oral steroids may be necessary

  The inflammation is self-limiting and the thyroid gland usually recovers with or without a brief period of hypothyroidism.

What are the causes of thyrotoxicosis?

The causes of thyrotoxicosis are listed in Table 29.

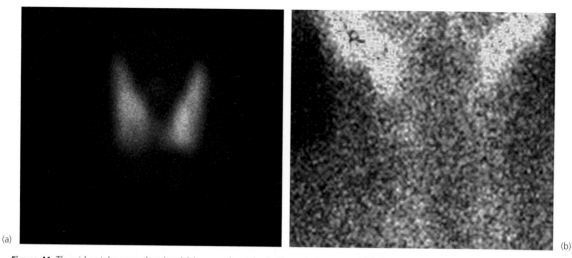

(a)   (b)

Figure 41 Thyroid uptake scan showing (a) increased uptake in Graves' disease and (b) decreased uptake in a case of thyroiditis.

Table 29 The aetiology of thyrotoxicosis.

Associated with increased thyroid hormone production by thyroid cells	Not associated with increased thyroid hormone production by thyroid cells
Graves' disease (80% of cases of thyrotoxicosis)	Thyroiditis (de Quervain's, postpartum thyroiditis, following amiodarone treatment)
Toxic nodule or toxic multinodular goitre	
TSH-secreting pituitary tumour	Exogenous thyroid hormone use
Trophoblastic tumour secreting human chorionic gonadotrophin (hCG) with TSH-like activity	Production of thyroid hormones from ectopic thyroid tissue (Struma ovarii: a teratoma in the ovary producing thyroid hormones)
Pituitary thyroid hormone resistance (lack of negative feedback on TSH secretion)	

Box 18 Graves' disease during pregnancy

- Remission of Graves' disease is frequently seen in pregnancy and the dose of antithyroid drugs can be reduced and often stopped altogether (usually in the third trimester)
- Propylthiouracil, rather than carbimazole, is used during pregnancy, as some reports suggest a link between carbimazole use in pregnancy and rare congenital defects in the newborn, although this is not fully proven

What are the main points in relation to long-term treatment of this condition?

- Achieve euthyroidism
  - Medical treatment: a course of 6–18 months of antithyroid treatment can be given, which results in remission of 50% of Graves' disease patients. Antithyroid drugs do not induce disease remission in hyperthyroidism due to other causes
  - Radioactive iodine treatment is an effective treatment but commonly results in hypothyroidism. RAI should not be given to patients with active eye disease

○ Surgery is a treatment option, particularly in individuals with large goitres or in those who could not tolerate medical treatment

• Patients with Graves' disease should be monitored for the occurrence of extrathyroidal complications

---

Box 19 Treatment of thyroid storm

• A thyroid storm is a rare but life-threatening complication of severe hyperthyroidism
• It can be precipitated by:
  ○ Infection
  ○ Surgery
  ○ Radiographic contrast agents
  ○ Withdrawal of antithyroid treatment
• Clinical manifestations include:
  ○ Confusion
  ○ High fever
  ○ Signs of severe hyperthyroidism (including tachyarrhythmias)

  ○ Multisystem failure (heart, lung, kidney and liver)
• Management
  ○ Patient should be transferred to intensive care and a senior endocrinologist should be involved in the management
  ○ Treat dehydration, arrhythmias and infection
  ○ Give high-dose propylthiouracil via nasogastric tube
  ○ Give β-blockers (preferably propranolol) as an infusion
  ○ Cover with high-dose steroids
  ○ Potassium iodide may be used, after starting antithyroid drugs, to inhibit thyroid hormone release

---

CASE REVIEW

Andrea, who is 35 years old, consults her doctor with a short history of palpitations, weakness and irritability. On further questioning, it becomes apparent that she has a number of symptoms suggestive of hyperthyroidism including heat intolerance, hand tremor and insomnia. On examination, she is found to have a hand tremor, sweaty palms and lid lag further suggesting hyperthyroidism. A raised T3 (requested after finding normal T4 levels) with suppressed TSH confirms hyperthyroidism. A diagnosis of Graves' disease is made, supported by the presence of a smooth goitre and eye changes (Graves' ophthalmopathy or thyroid-associated ophthalmopathy). In unclear cases, thyrotropin receptor antibodies can be requested, which are positive in more than 95% of Graves' patients, whereas thyroid peroxidase antibodies are positive in around 80%.

Treatment of Graves' disease includes antithyroid drugs, radioactive iodine and surgery, and these options should be discussed with the patients. A rare, and potentially fatal, side effect of antithyroid drugs is agranulocytosis, and all patients should be warned of the possibility of this complication.

Jill, Andrea's friend, also has classical symptoms of thyrotoxicosis with no clear goitre or eye signs but the neck is tender to palpation. Also, her symptoms started following a viral illness, raising the possibility of thyroiditis as a cause. This is further supported by negative thyrotropin antibodies and the diagnosis is confirmed by demonstrating the absence of technetium uptake on thyroid scan. Treatment of this condition is symptomatic (β-blockers, pain killers and rarely a short course of steroids).

KEY POINTS

• Hyperthyroidism is a common condition, affecting mainly the female population, and Graves' disease is the underlying aetiology in 80% of cases. Other causes of hyperthyroidism include toxic nodule or toxic multinodular goitre and thyroiditis
• Hyperthyroidism due to Graves' disease can be associated with extrathyroidal complications, including Graves' ophthalmopathy and pretibial myxoedema

• The commonest symptoms of hyperthyroidism include: heat intolerance, hand tremor, palpitations, frequent bowel motions, irritability and weight loss despite an increase in appetite. However, some individuals, particularly the elderly, can present with non-specific symptoms (apathetic hyperthyroidism)
• Treatments for hyperthyroidism include:
  ○ Antithyroid drugs: result in remission of hyperthyroidism

Continued

due to Graves' disease in around half of individuals. Hyperthyroidism due to other causes usually relapses after stopping antithyroid drugs. Antithyroid drugs may cause agranulocytosis and patients should be warned about the possibility of developing this serious, but fortunately rare, complication

- ○ Radioactive iodine: one dose of radioactive iodine is effective at controlling hyperthyroidism in the majority of patients, but hypothyroidism and long-term thyroxine replacement is a likely complication. This treatment should be avoided in pregnant women, individuals with urinary incontinence, patients with active eye disease and children (the latter is not an absolute contraindication)
- ○ Surgery: reserved for those with personal preference, active eye disease with intolerance to medical treatment, large disfiguring goitres and fears of malignancy

- A prompt referral to an ophthalmology assessment is required in patients with GO if they experience:
- ○ Decrease in visual acuity
- ○ Problems with colour vision
- ○ Inability to fully close the eyelids (leaving the sclerae exposed)
- ○ Sudden ophthalmoplegia

John, who is a 61-year-old postman, presents to his GP with a 6-week history of increasing tiredness, polyuria and polydipsia. He also noticed weight loss over the past 6 months (around 5 kg) and an irritating cough that seems to have coincided with him stopping smoking around 5 months ago. His past medical history includes a partial gastrectomy for a gastric ulcer 26 years ago, which according to John was related to heavy alcohol intake. He was a heavy smoker (40/day) for 38 years, but stopped 5 months ago due to increasing shortness of breath.

What is the differential diagnosis at this stage? What is the next step?

John presents with a 6-week history of polyuria and polydipsia, the differential diagnosis of which includes:
- Electrolyte abnormalities such as hypercalcaemia
- Chronic renal disease
- Diabetes insipidus
- Osmotic diuresis due to high plasma glucose levels (diabetes mellitus)
- The use of drugs such as lithium and demeclocycline
    The rest of the medical history includes:
- Recent weight loss
- Cough and increasing breathlessness
- A history of previous heavy smoking

    The history of smoking, respiratory symptoms and weight loss, should raise the suspicion of lung malignancy. Polyuria and polydipsia may be due to hypercalcaemia, which can be associated with malignancy (hypercalcaemia of malignancy). The next step is full examination, with special emphasis on the respiratory system.

On examination, John looks dehydrated, has a temperature of 36.6°C, blood pressure of 130/75, pulse 92 beats/min

regular, and respiratory rate 22 breaths/min. A 3.5-cm mass can be felt in the left clavicular fossa. Chest examination shows dullness to percussion, reduced breath sounds and vocal fremitus on the left side. Abdominal examination is unremarkable.

Does this help in making the diagnosis?

The patient has signs compatible with a left pleural effusion, a common finding in lung malignancy. Also, there is a large mass in the supraclavicular fossa, which may be due to lymph node metastasis from a primary lung cancer.

What tests would you request in this patient?

- FBC: anaemia is commonly associated with malignant conditions. Pancytopenia can be seen with marrow invasion by the tumour (advanced metastatic stage)
- U&Es: the patient is clinically dehydrated and hypercalcaemia of malignancy can impair renal function. Also, U&Es should be checked in patients with polyuria and polydipsia
- Calcium: malignancy can be associated with hypercalcaemia and its presence would explain the polyuria and polydipsia in this patient
- Glucose: this should be checked in any patient with polyuria and polydipsia to rule out the possibility of diabetes
- LFTs: abnormal LFTs may indicate liver metastasis in a patient with suspected malignancy. However, normal liver function does not rule out liver metastasis
- CXR: to investigate the abnormal physical findings

Tests showed:
FBC: Hb 9.8 g/L, WBC 6.7× 10⁹/L, platelets 365× 10⁹/L
U&Es: Na 145 mmol/L, K 3.6 mmol/L, urea 15.1 mmol/L, creatinine 192 μmol/L
Calcium: 2.8 mmol/L, corrected 3.2 mmol/L (normal range 2.1–2.6)

Endocrinology and Diabetes: Clinical Cases Uncovered. By R. Ajjan. Published 2009 by Blackwell Publishing, ISBN: 978-1-4051-5726-1

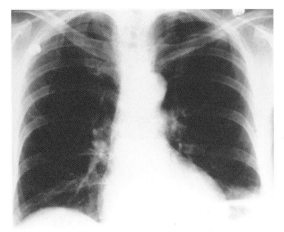

Figure 42

Random glucose: 5.6 mmol/L
LFTs (normal ranges):
    ALT 110 U/L (8–40)
    AP 465 U/L (36–200)
    Bilirubin 34 umol/L (4–18)
    Albumin 25 g/L (30–50)
CXR (see Fig. 42)

Comment on these results. What other blood test would you request?

These results show:

• FBC: mild anaemia, which is commonly seen in malignant conditions

• U&Es: deranged renal function probably related, at least in part, to dehydration secondary to hypercalcaemia

• Corrected calcium is elevated. It should be noted that calcium levels should always be adjusted according to albumin levels, as uncorrected calcium may underestimate hypercalcaemia in subjects with low albumin

• Deranged LFTs suggest liver metastasis and this should be further investigated with appropriate imaging techniques

• CXR: a left pleural effusion consistent with the clinical findings

Parathyroid hormone (PTH) plasma levels should be requested in any individual with raised plasma calcium to rule out the possibility of primary hyperparathyroidism. In hypercalcaemia of malignancy, PTH is undetectable, whereas in primary hyperparathyroidism PTH is high or in the high normal range.

What are the causes of hypercalcaemia? What is the aetiology of hypercalcaemia of malignancy?

Causes of hypercalcaemia include:

1 Excessive bone resorption
   ○ Primary hyperparathyroidism: relatively common condition, diagnosed by the presence of hypercalcaemia with elevated plasma PTH levels
   ○ Hypercalcaemia of malignancy without bony metastasis: due to the production PTH-related peptides (which mimic the action of PTH)
   ○ Hypercalcaemia of malignancy with bony metastasis: bone destruction resulting in hypercalcaemia
   ○ Hyperthyroidism: a rare cause of 'mild' hypercalcaemia

2 Excessive gastrointestinal calcium absorption
   ○ Milk-alkali syndrome
   ○ Vitamin D toxicity
   ○ Granulomatous disorders such as sarcoidosis

3 Increased renal reabsorption of calcium
   ○ Thiazide diuretic use: these are associated with hypocalciuria, which may result in mild hypercalcaemia
   ○ Familial hypocalciuric hypercalcaemia: an autosomal dominant condition due to a mutation in the calcium-sensing receptor. Diagnosis is made by demonstrating low urinary calcium excretion (in primary hyperparathyroidism, urinary calcium excretion is high)

4 Uncertain mechanisms
   ○ Addison's disease

The mechanisms of hypercalcaemia of malignancy include:

• Tumour secretion of PTH-related peptide (PTHrP) that mimics the action of PTH

• Bony destruction due to metastases to the bone, consequently releasing the calcium into the blood stream

How would you treat John's endocrine problem?

• Fluid replacement is the first step in the treatment of hypercalcaemia due to any cause, and usually large amounts are required (3–6 L of 0.9% saline over the first 24 h)

• Once the patient is volume replete, intravenous bisphosphonates can be used, which are very effective at correcting clinically significant hypercalcaemia. Pamidronate is most frequently used at doses of 30–90 mg diluted in 0.9% saline

• Calcitonin can also be used to treat hypercalcaemia, which is usually reserved for patients not responding to bisphosphonate

• High-dose steroids may be necessary to treat some resistant cases of hypercalcaemia of malignancy

CASE REVIEW

John, a 61-year-old postman, presents with a few weeks' history of tiredness, polyuria and polydipsia. Other complaints include significant weight loss and a cough that coincided with him stopping smoking (used to smoke 40/day for almost 40 years) around 5 months ago due to shortness of breath. The differential diagnosis of polyuria and polydipsia should be kept in mind and an appropriate history taken. Weight loss and cough in a smoker should always raise the suspicion of lung malignancy. On examination, John was dehydrated and a mass was palpable in the supraclavicular fossa. Chest auscultation was consistent with a left pleural effusion. Taken together, lung

malignancy is a strong probability and the osmotic symptoms may be due to hypercalcaemia of malignancy, frequently seen with advanced cancers. Blood tests confirm hypercalcaemia, in addition to abnormal liver function, which may be due to metastatic disease. From the endocrine point of view, John will need to be rehydrated first and then treated with bisphosphonate infusion to control his hypercalcaemia. Longer term, appropriate management of the lung condition should help to correct his hypercalcaemia but repeated bisphosphonate and even steroid therapy may also be required.

KEY POINTS

• Hypercalcaemia is a common condition and should be suspected in individuals with:
  ○ Osmotic symptoms (polyuria, polydipsia)
  ○ Abdominal pain
  ○ Constipation
• Causes of hypercalcaemia include:
  ○ Primary hyperparathyroidism (common) and tertiary hyperparathyroidism (renal failure patients, rare)
  ○ Hypercalcaemia of malignancy
  ○ Dietary (milk alkali syndrome)
  ○ Drugs (thiazides)

  ○ Hypocalciuric hypocalcaemia (should be suspected in the presence of family history of hypercalcaemia)
• Treatments for hypercalcaemia include:
  ○ Treat the cause
  ○ In severe symptomatic hypercalcaemia (commonly due to malignancy), management includes: intravenous rehydration, intravenous bisphosphonate and sometimes steroids (the latter can be effective in resistant hypercalcaemia of malignancy)
• Complications of long-term untreated hypercalcaemia include renal calculi, nephrocalcinosis and renal failure

Case 4 A 44-year-old woman with visual problems

Debra, a 44-year-old woman, is seen by her optician for recent deterioration of her vision. The optician performs a visual field test, results of which are shown in Fig. 43.

What abnormality can you see?
The visual field test shows bilateral hemianopia.

Where is the lesion?
The lesion is at the optic chiasm. The different types of visual field defects are shown in Fig. 44.

What pathology does the above lesion suggest?
This suggests a pathology in the pituitary gland such as a pituitary tumour growing outside the pituitary fossa and causing compression of the optic chiasm.

What questions would you ask?
A pituitary tumour may be associated with increased production of a pituitary hormone or may be a non-functioning tumour. Large tumours may result in reduced production of one or multiple hormones due to compressive effects on normal pituitary cells, and may also result in cranial nerve palsies due to invasion of the cavernous sinus. Therefore, the questions to ask would concern the following symptoms:

- Excessive production of prolactin (prolactinoma):
  ○ Galactorrhoea (90% of women, 10% of men)
  ○ Menstrual irregularities
  ○ Low libido and impotence
- Excessive secretion of growth hormone (acromegaly):
  ○ Change in glove or shoe size
  ○ Excessive sweating
  ○ Arthralgia, headaches
  ○ Symptoms of diabetes

- Excessive secretion of ACTH (Cushing's disease):
  ○ Weight gain
  ○ Easy bruising
  ○ Proximal muscle weakness
  ○ Mood disturbance
  ○ Menstrual irregularities
  ○ Low libido and impotence
  ○ Recurrent infections
  ○ Symptoms of diabetes
- Excessive production of TSH (TSH-oma): symptoms of hyperthyroidism as detailed in Case 2
- Excessive production of FSH or LH: these are rare and usually present in the same manner as a non-functioning pituitary adenoma

If none of the above symptoms is present, then we are probably dealing with a non-functioning adenoma, which, if large enough, may cause compression of healthy pituitary tissue resulting in a variable degree of pituitary insufficiency. Therefore, symptoms of hormonal deficiency should be considered including:

- Growth hormone deficiency
  ○ Tiredness
  ○ Impaired psychological well-being
- ACTH
  ○ Symptoms of primary hypoadrenalism, except for the lack of pigmentation
- TSH
  ○ Symptoms of primary hypothyroidism
- FSH/LH
  ○ Menstrual irregularities
  ○ Reduced libido and erectile dysfunction in men

What signs would you look for during examination of Debra?
- Prolactinoma
  ○ Galactorrhoea
- Acromegaly
  ○ Coarse facial appearance (prognathism, increased

Endocrinology and Diabetes: Clinical Cases Uncovered. By R. Ajjan.
Published 2009 by Blackwell Publishing, ISBN: 978-1-4051-5726-1

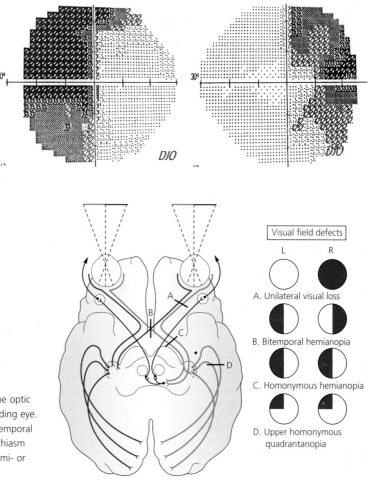

Figure 43 Results of visual field testing.

Figure 44 Visual field defect. A. lesion in the optic nerve causes loss of vision in the corresponding eye. B. lesion in the optic chiasm results in a bitemporal field defect. C,D. lesion distal to the optic chiasm may result in contralateral homonymous hemi- or quadrantanopia.

dental separation, frontal bossing, oily skin, tongue enlargement
  ○ Deep voice
  ○ Enlargement of hands and feet
  ○ Soft tissue swelling (may result in carpal tunnel syndrome)
  ○ Organomegaly
  ○ Hypertension,
• Cushing's disease:
  ○ Facial appearance (round and plethoric face, acne and hirsutism)
  ○ Truncal obesity with thin extremities
  ○ Thin and fragile skin
  ○ Hypertension
  ○ Osteoporosis (may cause vertebral fracture)
• TSH-secreting tumour
  ○ Signs of hyperthyroidism

Fig. 45 is an MRI of Debra's brain. It shows a large pituitary tumour causing compression of the optic chiasm, and, hence, the visual field defect.

What tests would you request to rule out hormonal excess or deficiencies?

Tests for hormonal excess include:
• Prolactinoma: plasma prolactin levels
• Acromegaly: glucose tolerance test. Administration of glucose suppresses growth hormone production and failure of this suppression is strongly suggestive of acromegaly
• Cushing's disease: dexamethasone suppression test. Administration of dexamethasone results in suppression of cortisol production. Failure of suppression indicates Cushing's syndrome, which may be due to Cushing's

disease, ectopic ACTH production or excessive production of cortisol by an adrenal tumour
• TSH-secreting tumour: TFTs. Thyroid hormones will be elevated and, in contrast to primary hyperthyroidism, TSH will also be elevated

Tests for pituitary hormone deficiency include:
• TFTs (assess thyroid hormone status)
• Glucagon stimulation test or insulin stress test (assess growth hormone and pituitary adrenal axis)

Tests for hormonal deficiencies are not required if the patient is scheduled for emergency surgery. The patient will be covered with steroid during the operation and tests for hormonal deficiencies will be done routinely after the surgical procedure as surgery itself may result in damage to normal pituitary tissue, consequently resulting in hypopituitarism.

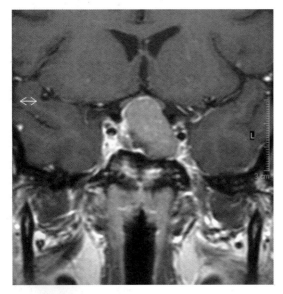

Figure 45

Debra has no symptoms or signs of hormonal excess or deficiency.

What one endocrine blood test would you request that may have important implications for the clinical management in this case?

• It is important to exclude a prolactinoma (raised prolactin levels), which may be clinically silent (except for the local effect), particularly in men
• The management of prolactinomas is usually medical, and, therefore, patients can be spared surgical intervention
• However, large non-functioning tumours may cause raised prolactin due to stalk compression, but prolactin in this case is usually less than 6000 mU/L. In contrast, in large pituitary macroprolactinoma (the term 'macro' defines tumours >1 cm in diameter) prolactin levels are usually >10 000 mU/L and can even exceed 100 000 mU/L

Provided all her hormonal tests are normal, what is the diagnosis and best treatment option?

• The most likely diagnosis here is a large non-functioning pituitary adenoma
• The best treatment option is surgical removal (usually transphenoidal surgery)

One day after the initial assessment, Debra attends A&E with severe headaches, double vision, dizziness and vomiting.

What does Fig. 46 show and what is the diagnosis?

• Fig. 46 shows complete right ptosis, abduction of the right eye with mydriasis (dilated pupil)
• The diagnosis is right third nerve palsy

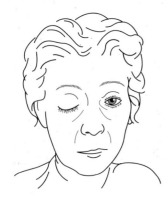
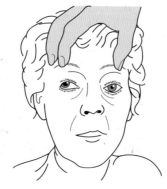

Figure 46

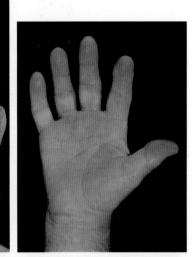

Figure 5 Typical acromegalic facial features. Courtesy of Dr Steve Orme.

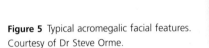

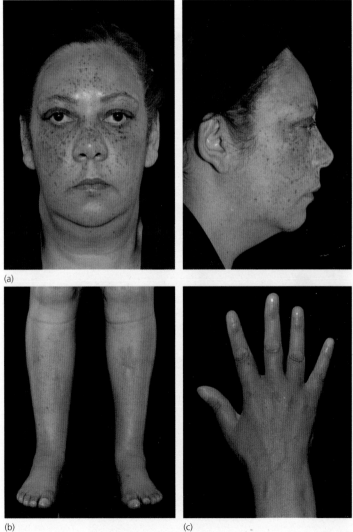

(a)

(b)

(c)

Figure 9 Extrathyroidal manifestations of Graves' disease. (a) Graves' ophthalmopathy showing proptosis and previous tarsorrhaphy in a patient with inactive disease. (b) Quiescent myxoedema, secondary to the accumulation of glycosaminoglycans and associated inflammatory infiltrate. (c) Graves' acropachy, which looks similar to clubbing and is due to subperiostal new bone formation.

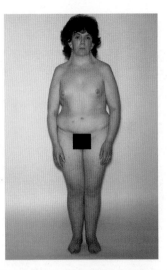

Figure 25 Characteristics of Turner's syndrome; short stature, webbed neck, poor breast development and widely spaced nipples. Courtesy of Dr Paul Belchetz.

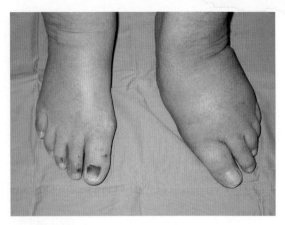

Figure 29 Deformed, red and hot ankle joint in a diabetes subject should raise the suspicion of Charcot's osteoarthropathy. Diagnosis can be confirmed by X-rays (these can be normal in the early stages), magnetic resonance imaging and isotope bone scans. Courtesy of Dr Carol Amery.

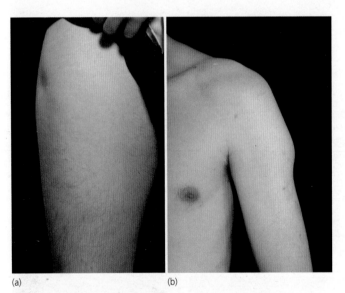

(a)　　　　　　　　　　　(b)

Figure 35 Potential complications at insulin injection sites. (a) Lipoatrophy and (b) lipohypertrophy at insulin injection sites

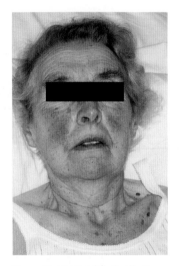

Figure 38 Carcinoid flush affecting the face. Courtesy of Dr Paul Belchetz.

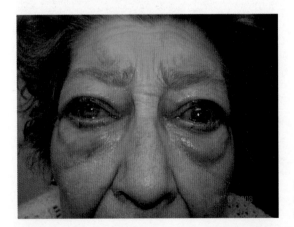

Figure 40 Periorbital oedema, conjunctival infection, chemosis and proptosis in an individual with active Graves' ophthalmopathy. Courtesy of Mr Bernard Chang.

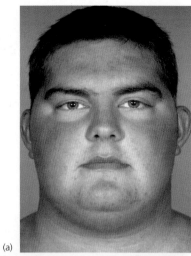

(a)

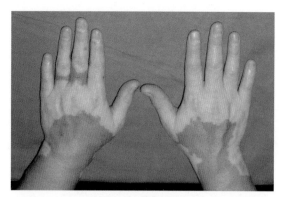

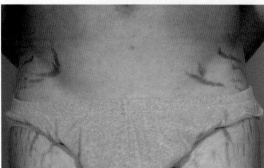

(b)

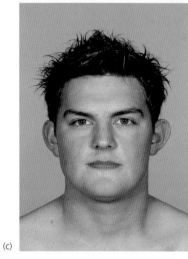

(c)

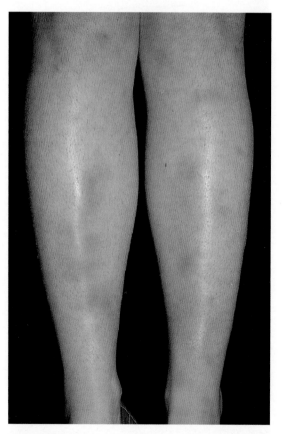

Figure 47 Cushing's disease (a), (b) before treatment, (c) after treatment. Courtesy of Dr Dinesh Nagi.

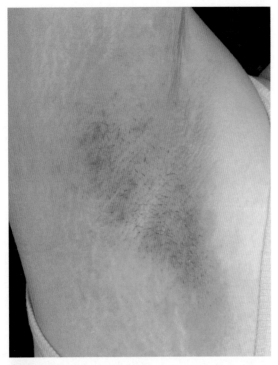

Figure 56

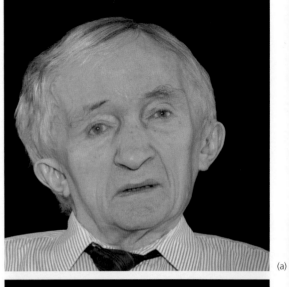

(a)

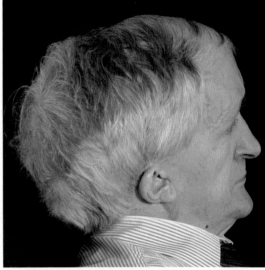

(b)

Figure 60 (a, b) Paget's disease of the skull.

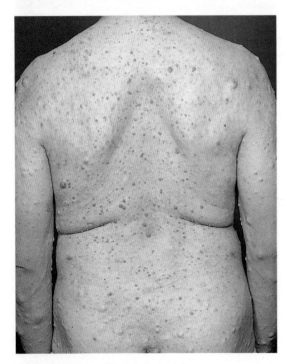

Figure 62 Courtesy of Dr D.A. Burns, Leicester.

What complication has occurred? How would the patient present and what test would you request?

- The most likely diagnosis is pituitary apoplexy (pituitary infarction)
- The patient typically presents with sudden onset headache, vomiting, visual disturbances and cranial nerve palsies
- Diagnosis is based on typical MRI findings, which should be requested urgently

What urgent medical management does she need? What other treatment can be offered?

- Pituitary apoplexy is usually associated with cessation of pituitary hormone production due to infarction in the pituitary tissue. This results in low ACTH levels, consequently leading to inadequate cortisol production by the adrenal gland, which may result in a hypoadrenal crisis.

Therefore, urgent medical treatment with intravenous cortisol is required in patients with suspected pituitary apoplexy. Low levels of other hormones are less critical short term, and these can be replaced later
- Neurosurgeons should be informed as these patients are usually treated with early surgical intervention; however, some are managed conservatively if there are no visual or neurological symptoms

How and where should patients with previous pituitary tumours be followed up?

Individuals with pituitary pathology should always be followed up in specialized centres to monitor:
- Recurrence of the disease
- Check for the development of complete/partial pituitary failure (particularly those who had pituitary radiotherapy)
- Ensure adequate hormonal replacement

CASE REVIEW

Debra, a middle-aged woman, is seen by her optician for recent deterioration of her vision. Her visual field testing shows bitemporal hemianopia suggesting a lesion in the optic chiasm, possibly secondary to a pituitary pathology. An appropriate history focussing on excess or deficient pituitary hormone production should be taken in any individual with suspected pituitary tumour. In this case, there are no clear indications for pituitary hormone excess or deficiency and Debra undergoes an MRI scan, which shows a large pituitary tumour compressing the optic chiasm. It is important to rule out the possibility of prolactinoma (which responds to medical treatment);

Debra's endocrine tests are normal suggesting she has a non-functioning pituitary adenoma, for which surgical intervention is the best treatment option. Debra suddenly develops severe headaches and third nerve palsy, associated with dizziness and vomiting. In view of the large pituitary tumour, pituitary apoplexy (infarction) is a strong possibility, which is a known complication of pituitary tumours. Neurosurgeons should be informed of the latest development, an urgent MRI requested and the patient should be covered with steroids (due to potential loss of ACTH-secreting cells).

KEY POINTS

- Pituitary tumours may be non-functioning or functional secreting one or more of pituitary hormones
- Individuals with bitemporal hemianopia should be suspected as having a pituitary tumour. On the other hand, pituitary tumours may occur without visual field defects if the tumour is not compressing the optic chiasm
- Individuals with pituitary tumours should be assessed both clinically and biochemically for pituitary hormone excess. They should also be assessed for pituitary hormone deficiency and possible cranial nerve pathologies
- The commonest functional pituitary tumour is a

prolactinoma, which is unique amongst the pituitary tumours as it can be treated medically without the need for surgery in the majority of patients
- Following surgery, patients should be checked for pituitary hormonal deficiencies using appropriate tests
- Long-term monitoring for pituitary failure is warranted for patients who have had pituitary radiotherapy (for recurrent or incompletely resected pituitary tumours)
- All pituitary patients should be followed up long term in specialized centres to monitor disease recurrence, development of pituitary failure and ensure adequate hormone replacement

Case 5   A 20-year-old man with recent diagnosis of diabetes

Richard, a 20-year-old man, is referred to the diabetes clinic with newly diagnosed diabetes (fasting glucose on two occasions >10 mmol/L). He has had osmotic symptoms (polyuria and polydipsia) for at least 6 months and his weight has recently increased by around 14 kg. Fig. 47a,b (colour plate section) shows Richard's face and abdomen.

What do you see?
- The face appears round (moon-like)
- There is truncal obesity and abdominal striae

What questions would you like to ask Richard? What signs would you look for?
Questions should be asked to look for evidence of:
- Easy bruising
- Muscle weakness
- Mood disturbances
- Low libido and impotence
  Signs to look for include:
- Thin skin with easy bruising
- Proximal muscle weakness
- Hypertension

Richard is unable to stand from a squatting position, has very thin skin with multiple bruising and is hypertensive at 160/95 mmHg.

Does Richard have type 1 or type 2 diabetes? Why?
Neither. Richard has a secondary form of diabetes as a complication of Cushing's syndrome. Richard has classical features of Cushing's syndrome including:
- Facial appearance (round 'moon-like' face)
- Truncal obesity and abdominal striae
- Thin skin and easy bruising

Endocrinology and Diabetes: Clinical Cases Uncovered. By R. Ajjan. Published 2009 by Blackwell Publishing, ISBN: 978-1-4051-5726-1

- Proximal muscle weakness (hence inability to stand from a squatting position).
- Complications of the disease:
  ○ Diabetes
  ○ Hypertension
  The clinical features of Cushing's syndrome are summarized in Table 30.

What are the aetiologies of Cushing's syndrome and what tests would you request here to confirm the diagnosis?
Cushing's syndrome may be due to:
1. Pituitary adenoma secreting excessive ACTH (Cushing's disease)
2. Ectopic ACTH secretion due to a malignant tumour secreting ACTH
3. Adrenal tumour secreting excessive cortisol
4. Cushing's syndrome secondary to exogenous steroid use (patients treated with steroids for, e.g. respiratory problems and rheumatoid arthritis)

Tests to diagnose Cushing's syndrome include (detailed in Part 1, p. 31):
- Midnight cortisol
- Overnight dexamethasone suppression test
- Low-dose dexamethasone suppression test
- 24-h urinary cortisol

Once a diagnosis of Cushing's syndrome has been made, further tests should be done to establish the aetiology.
- A good clinical history can quickly exclude Cushing's syndrome secondary to exogenous steroids
- To differentiate between 1, 2 and 3, ACTH should be measured which is elevated in 1 and 2, whereas it is undetectable in 3 (excessive cortisol results in suppression of pituitary ACTH secretion)
- Differentiating between 1 and 2 can be more difficult:
  ○ A low potassium is suggestive of ectopic ACTH production (hypokalaemia is found in 90%), but it is not diagnostic as 10% of Cushing's disease patients may have hypokalaemia

Table 30 Symptoms and signs of Cushing's syndrome.

Symptoms	Signs
Weight gain	Facial appearance: round face, acne and hirsutism
Truncal obesity	Central obesity and abdominal striae
Easy bruising	Thin skin and easy bruising
Muscle weakness	Proximal muscle weakness
Mood disturbances (depression, psychosis)	Hypertension
Menstrual irregularities	Impaired glucose tolerance or diabetes
Low libido and impotence	Fractures due to osteoporosis
Recurrent infections	Vascular disease

○ High-dose dexamethasone suppression test: in pituitary Cushing's cortisol levels fall by >50% of basal values. However, in a minority of ectopic ACTH-secreting tumours, cortisol can be also suppressed by more than 50% of basal values

○ Inferior petrosal sampling may be necessary to measure levels of ACTH after corticotrophin releasing hormone stimulation in the inferior petrosal sinus. High central (in the petrosal sinus) to peripheral (peripheral vein) ACTH levels are diagnostic of Cushing's disease

If a diagnosis of ectopic ACTH is made, investigations should focus on finding the tumour secreting excessive ACTH.

What are the treatment options for Cushing's disease?

• Transphenoidal surgery is the best treatment but is not always successful

• Radiotherapy can be used as a second-line treatment following:
  ○ Relapsed disease
  ○ Unsuccessful surgery
• Medical treatment is indicated in:
  ○ The perioperative period
  ○ Patients in whom surgery is contraindicated
  ○ While awaiting radiotherapy to take effect (which may take months to years)
  ○ Drugs used include: metyrapone and ketoconazole
• Adrenalectomy: this is usually reserved for cases not responsive to the above treatment measures

What is cyclical Cushing's?

A minority of Cushing's syndrome patients have intermittent cortisol secretion, which can make the life of the investigating endocrinologist very difficult indeed. The results of the dynamic tests can only be accurately interpreted when the disease is clinically active, and, therefore, repeated investigations are required.

Box 20 Complications of Cushing's disease

• Hypertension
• Impaired glucose tolerance/diabetes
• Osteoporosis
• Susceptibility to infection
• Easy bruising due to thin and fragile skin

Other complications vary according to the aetiology of the disease. For example, patients with Cushing's disease may have complications related to the pituitary mass (visual field defect, pituitary apoplexy). Patients with ectopic ACTH secretion may develop complications secondary to the presence of a malignant tumour (e.g. haemoptysis from a primary lung tumour or complications arising secondary to metastasis).

CASE REVIEW

Richard is a young man who presents with new diagnosis of diabetes and significant weight gain. He has evidence of excessive steroid hormone production (Cushing's syndrome) manifested as a round and 'moon-like' face, central obesity with abdominal striae, thin skin, easy bruising, hypertension and proximal muscle weakness. Cushing's syndrome can be due to increased ACTH production by a pituitary tumour or by non-pituitary malignant tissue (ectopic ACTH secretion), both of which are associated with increased plasma ACTH levels. In

Continued

contrast, Cushing's syndrome due to an adrenal adenoma or exogenous steroid administration are associated with suppression of ACTH production.

Tests to diagnose Cushing's syndrome include midnight cortisol, overnight dexamethasone suppression test, low-dose dexamethasone suppression test and 24-h urinary cortisol. Differentiation between causes of Cushing's syndrome can be difficult and requires specialist input. Complications of Cushing's syndrome include hypertension, diabetes, increased susceptibility to infections and osteoporosis. Treatment of Cushing's syndrome depends on the aetiology of the condition and medical therapy with metyrapone or ketoconazole can be considered until definitive treatment measures are used.

KEY POINTS

- Cushing's syndrome is a condition that arises secondary to increased plasma cortisol levels
- Cushing's syndrome can be:
  - ACTH-dependent, e.g. pituitary tumours and ectopic ACTH production by malignant tissue
  - Non-ACTH dependent, e.g. adrenal adenoma and prolonged, high-dose steroid treatment (for asthma, rheumatoid arthritis, etc.)
- The main clinical features of Cushing's syndrome include:
  - Round, 'moon-like' face
  - Weight gain, central obesity and abdominal striae
  - Thin skin and easy bruising
  - Proximal muscle weakness
  - Hypertension and vascular disease
  - Diabetes
  - Increased susceptibility to infections
  - Fractures due to osteoporosis
- Biochemical tests for the diagnosis of Cushing's syndrome include:
  - Midnight cortisol
  - Overnight or low-dose dexamethasone suppression test
  - Urinary cortisol (collection over 24 h)
- Treatment of Cushing's syndrome differs according to the aetiology of the condition

Tiredness and weight gain in a 30-year-old woman with diabetes

PART 2: CASES

Iwona is a 30-year-old woman with known type 1 diabetes for 12 years. She visits her GP complaining of tiredness and weight gain. Her HbA1c levels over the past 7 years have ranged between 6.4 and 7.1%, but her most recent test showed an HbA1c of 8.3%.

What would you do at this stage?

This is a young woman with type 1 diabetes that has been well controlled indicating that she is a reliable and a compliant patient. Her diabetes control has deteriorated recently, which may be related to:

• Weight gain
• Change in the dose of insulin
• Compliance issues
• Problems with the injection sites (i.e. lipohypertrophy)
• Weight gain may be due to:
   ◦ Change in lifestyle (different diet, less exercise)
   ◦ Endocrine problems (Cushing's syndrome, hypothyroidism)
   ◦ Depression (some individuals with depression tend to eat more)
• Tiredness is a non-specific symptom (reviewed elsewhere). In this particular patient, it may simply be due to deterioration in diabetes control

A more detailed history at this stage is essential, in particular addressing any change in diet, lifestyle or dose of insulin.

Iwona tells you that her diet has not changed but she is undertaking less exercise due to extreme fatigue. The dose of her insulin has not changed and she continues in her current job as a teacher and has no family problems or social issues of note.

Endocrinology and Diabetes: Clinical Cases Uncovered. By R. Ajjan. Published 2009 by Blackwell Publishing, ISBN: 978-1-4051-5726-1

How does this information help you?

• The above suggests that Iwona has an organic cause for her tiredness that is probably not directly related to her diabetes
• Her symptoms should be further explored keeping in mind the association of type 1 diabetes with other endocrine autoimmune conditions such as hypothyroidism and hypoadrenalism
• Hypothyroidism is a common disease, particularly in type 1 diabetes and questions regarding specific symptoms of hypothyroidism (Table 9, p. 18) should be asked at this stage
• The possibility of hypoadrenalism (Addison's disease) is less likely as this is usually associated with weight loss and hypoglycaemia (or reduced insulin requirements), which are not seen here

On further questioning, Iwona tells you that her skin is getting very dry, is feeling constantly cold and her hair is becoming coarse and brittle. Also, she has had recent problems with menstrual irregularities and has been constipated.

What would you do now?

Iwona's symptoms are consistent with hypothyroidism, and, therefore, examination of her thyroid status should be the next step (Part 1, p. 34).

On examination, Iwona indeed has dry skin and inspection of her face reveals periorbital puffiness. Her pulse is slow at 52 beats/min regular and she has slow relaxing reflexes. Neck palpation reveals no goitre.

What is your diagnosis so far and what tests would you request?

• Iwona has classical signs of hypothyroidism (summarized in Table 9, p. 18). Therefore, the likely diagnosis is autoimmune hypothyroidism (AH), which may occur:

○ In the presence of a thyroid goitre, a goitrous form or Hashimoto's thyroiditis

○ In the absence of a thyroid goitre, the atrophic form or primary myxoedema

• The diagnosis can be confirmed by checking thyroid function tests (TFTs) and thyroid peroxidase (TPO) antibodies

○ TFTs are expected to show low thyroid hormones and raised TSH

○ TPO antibodies are usually positive in patients with AH

Iwona's tests show a FT4 of 6.1 mmol/L and TSH of 81 mIU/L with positive TPO antibodies.

How would you manage this patient now?

• These tests are consistent with AH and the patient will need T4 replacement therapy

• Thyroxine treatment can be started in a young patient at a full replacement dose. In the older age group, in those with cardiac problems, and in longstanding hypothyroidism, an initial small dose is advised with gradual titration to an appropriate maintenance dose

• TSH should be rechecked around 6 weeks after starting treatment or after modifying the dose of T4

• The maintenance dose of T4 is around 1.4 mcg/kg

Iwona tells you that she is planning a pregnancy in the next year or so.

What advice would you give her?

• Pregnant hypothyroid women usually need a 30–50% increase of T4 dose and this should be fully explained to patients with hypothyroidism of child-bearing age

• Iwona should inform her endocrinologist once she becomes pregnant, in order to increase the dose of T4 and make appropriate arrangements to monitor TFTs during pregnancy

Iwona's symptoms completely disappear on 100 mcg of T4, which is further increased to 150 mcg when she becomes pregnant 9 months later. She goes through an uneventful pregnancy and the dose of T4 is decreased after delivery to 100 mcg/day. Twelve months after delivery her TFTs showed a FT4 of 18.6 pmol/L and TSH 1.2 mU/L on 100 mcg T4.

What do these results indicate?

• The patient seems to be well replaced with thyroxine as both her FT4 and TSH are in the normal range

• It is advisable to have the TSH between 0.2 and 2.0 mU/L in patients having thyroxine replacement therapy, which is the case in this patient

Iwona comes to see you 2 years later complaining of tiredness, muscle cramps, aches and weight gain.

What would you do?

Iwona's TFTs should be checked as her symptoms are consistent with under-replacement with thyroxine.

Her TFTs showed:
FT4   22.1 pmol/L
TSH   15.8 mU/L

How do you explain these findings?

• This is a relatively common finding in patients on thyroxine replacement and is usually indicative of non-compliance

• The patient is not taking thyroxine regularly causing an elevation of TSH. However, the patient takes the thyroxine before the blood test resulting in normal FT4 but TSH remains high

○ It takes TSH a few weeks to normalize in patients having thyroxine replacement and this is why TFTs should not be repeated less than 4–6 weeks following initiation or change in treatment

Iwona admits to having some difficulties at work resulting in non-compliance. These issues are subsequently resolved and her TFTs normalize 3 months later.

She comes to see you again with a skin condition, as shown in Fig. 48 (colour plate section).

What is the diagnosis?

• Iwona's skin shows areas of decreased pigmentation

• The diagnosis is vitiligo

Is Iwona's skin condition related to her thyroid disease?

• Vitiligo is an autoimmune condition that can be associated with autoimmune disorders, particularly autoimmune thyroid disease

PART 2: CASES

Box 21 Causes of hypothyroidism

- Autoimmune thyroid disease
  - Non-goitrous: atrophic hypothyroidism
  - Goitrous: Hashimoto's thyroiditis
- Thyroiditis (including postpartum thyroiditis): hypothyroidism is usually preceded by a brief period of hyperthyroidism. It is a self-limiting disease and thyroid function usually normalizes, with or without a brief period of thyroxine treatment
- Drug-induced: amiodarone, lithium
- Post radiation or following treatment with radioactive iodine

- Congenital development and hereditary biosynthetic defects
- Iodine deficiency
- Thyroid surgery
- Secondary (lesion in the pituitary gland or hypothalamus)
- Thyroid hormone resistance (peripheral tissue fails to respond to thyroxine)
  See Table 9, p. 18 for symptoms and signs of hypothyroidism.

CASE REVIEW

Iwona is a young woman with known type 1 diabetes. She presents to her GP with classical symptoms of hypothyroidism including tiredness, weight gain, dry skin, cold intolerance, brittle hair and menstrual irregularities, in addition to deterioration in her glucose control. A diagnosis of autoimmune hypothyroidism is made by demonstrating low plasma FT4 with increased TSH and positive TPO antibodies. Her condition is successfully treated with thyroid hormone replacement. Subsequently, she becomes pregnant necessitating an increase in the dose of thyroxine, due to increased requirement of this hormone during pregnancy. Two years after giving birth, her blood test shows raised TSH with normal FT4, which turns out to be secondary to non-compliance, the commonest cause of such a blood abnormality in patients having thyroxine replacement.

KEY POINTS

- Hypothyroidism is a common condition, particularly in the presence of personal or family history of autoimmunity, and it affects mainly the female population
- The commonest aetiology is related to thyroid autoimmunity. Other causes include thyroiditis, medical treatment (amiodarone, lithium) and iodine deficiency
- Hypothyroidism can present with a wide range of clinical symptoms/signs, the commonest being:
  - Tiredness
  - Cold intolerance
  - Dry skin, brittle hair and puffy face
  - Weight gain
  - Constipation

  - Bradycardia
  - Slow-relaxing reflexes
  - Biochemical abnormalities in hypothyroidism include a raised TSH with low or low-normal FT4. Thyroid peroxidase antibodies are usually positive in hypothyroidism secondary to autoimmunity
  - Treatment of hypothyroidism is simple and involves thyroid hormone replacement, usually in the form of L-thyroxine (T4)
  - Dose of thyroxine usually needs adjustment during pregnancy or after weight gain/loss

Case 7   Acute confusion in an 82-year-old with known type 2 diabetes

Brian, an 82-year-old gentleman with known type 2 diabetes, is brought to A&E with general deterioration and acute confusion.

What differential diagnoses would you consider and what would you do?

Older people commonly present to hospital with acute and subacute confusional states. The differential diagnosis is wide and includes:

- Infection:
  - Urinary tract infections (UTIs), which are very common, particularly in women
  - Chest infections
  - Encephalitis and meningitis (rare)
- Drugs and alcohol
  - Intoxication (opiates, sedatives, anticholinergics)
  - Withdrawal
- Hypoxia
  - Central (sedatives)
  - Pulmonary (infection)
- Metabolic
  - Uraemia
  - Liver failure
  - Hypoglycaemia
  - Hypercalcaemia
- Vascular
  - Stroke
  - Transient ischaemic attack (TIA)
- Intracranial lesion:
  - Raised intracranial pressure (due to a brain tumour for example)
  - Subdural haematoma
- Epilepsy
  - Temporal lobe epilepsy
  - Post ictal states

- Nutritional deficiencies
  - B_{12}
  - Thiamine (particularly in alcoholics)

The first step is to take a proper history to narrow down the differential diagnosis. Questions asked should include:

- Onset of confusion
  - Acute
  - Acute on chronic
- Associated symptoms/previous history
  - Urinary symptoms or incontinence (UTI)
  - Cough or shortness of breath (chest infection)
  - Weakness in arms or legs or slurred speech (stroke/TIA)
  - Any falls (even mild head bumps may result in a subdural haematoma, particularly in patients treated with warfarin)
- History of alcohol abuse
- Detailed drug history

It is not possible to take a history from Brian as he is confused and agitated. Members of his family tell you that they saw Brian a week ago when he was absolutely fine. They stress that he is usually in good health and does his shopping and cooking and has been managing alone for 5 years after the death of his wife. Apart from diabetes and 'mild' hypertension, both diagnosed 10 years ago, he has never had any problems with his health. He drinks occasionally (1–4 units/month). His medications include:
Metformin 850 mg b.d.
Gliclazide 40 mg b.d.
Aspirin 75 mg o.d.
Atorvastatin 10 mg o.d.
Bendrofluazide 2.5 mg o.d.

Does this help you to rule out any of differential diagnoses mentioned above? What would you do next?

- Although limited, the history from the family estab-

Endocrinology and Diabetes: Clinical Cases Uncovered. By R. Ajjan. Published 2009 by Blackwell Publishing, ISBN: 978-1-4051-5726-1

lishes that this is an acute confusional state in an elderly gentleman who is managing to live alone with no apparent problems

• The list of Brian's medications does not include any sedatives or opiates and his alcohol intake is minimal, ruling out drugs/alcohol as a cause of his confusion. However, he is on gliclazide, which may cause hypoglycaemia. At this stage, an urgent test of capillary glucose is required

---

The nurse performs a set of initial assessments and these reveal:
Glasgow Coma Scale (GCS) 13/15 (E3, V5, M5)
Blood pressure 100/58
Pulse 110/min regular
Temperature 37.4°C
Respiratory rate 30/min
O2 saturation 89%
Capillary glucose 'high'

What would you do next?

• The patient is hypotensive and tachycardic with a drop in GCS

• He has low-grade temperature

• His oxygen saturation is low

• His capillary glucose is 'high' indicating blood sugar probably in excess of 30 mmol/L (most capillary glucose meters fail to accurately measure very high glucose levels and simply refer to these as 'high')

As Brian is tachypneic with low oxygen saturation, he should:

• Undergo a full physical examination with special emphasis on the respiratory system

• His arterial blood gases should be checked

• He should also be started on oxygen therapy

On examination, Brian is clinically dehydrated although cardiovascular and abdominal examination are both normal. Chest auscultation indicates decreased percussion note on the right with increased vocal fremitus and bronchial breathing. Neurological examination is difficult as the patient is uncooperative, but it is noted that he is: confused and agitated, moving all four limbs, his pupils are normal in size with a normal light reflex and plantars are down going.
Brian's arterial blood gas (ABG) analysis showed:
PO2 7.1 kPa
PCO2 2.3 kPa
HCO3 16 mmol/L
pH 7.32

What would you do next?

• The normal heart and abdominal examination make primary pathology in the cardiovascular and gastrointestinal system unlikely, although do not completely rule it out

• Although full neurological examination was difficult, the 'brief version' described above indicates that it is unlikely a major neurological pathology is causing the above abnormalities. However, this examination does not conclusively rule out a neurological condition. For example, a subdural haematoma does not necessarily cause any weakness and may manifest as unexplained confusion

• The respiratory examination is consistent with lung consolidation, making a diagnosis of pneumonia a strong possibility

• ABG analysis shows:
  ○ Hypoxia
  ○ Mild metabolic acidosis
  ○ Secondary hypocapnia (trying to correct the metabolic acidosis)

It is essential to test the urine for ketonuria in any diabetes patient with high blood glucose, particularly in the presence of acidosis, to rule out the possibility of diabetic ketoacidosis.

Brian's urine dipstick shows:
Glucose +++
Ketones +
WBC negative
Nitrates negative

Does Brian have DKA? What other conclusions can be made from the urine dipstick results?

• Brian's urine dipstick results are not compatible with DKA due to the absence of heavy ketonuria. Mild ketonuria can be frequently seen, particularly in fasted individuals

• The urine dipstick fails to show white cells or nitrates in the urine making a UTI an unlikely diagnosis

What other tests would you request in this patient?

• FBC: looking for raised white cells (infection), anaemia

• Blood cultures: raised temperature, likely chest infection

- U&Es: checking kidney function, particularly in view of the dehydration and acidosis
- Glucose: in view of the history of diabetes and raised capillary glucose
- CXR: in view of the positive findings on examination
- ECG: all acutely unwell individuals, particularly diabetes patients, should have an ECG done to rule out silent myocardial infarction and cardiac arrhythmias
- To complete the confusion screen, the following should be checked:
  ○ LFTs
  ○ Calcium
  ○ B_{12} plasma levels

What is the diagnosis so far and what would you do while awaiting the results of the above tests?

- In complicated cases, it is advisable to make a list of the abnormalities, which usually helps in organizing further investigations and reaching the correct diagnosis. The abnormalities in this case thus far:
  ○ Acute confusion
  ○ Signs of dehydration
  ○ Signs of chest infection
  ○ Hyperglycaemia
  ○ Hypoxia
  ○ Metabolic acidosis (mild, partially compensated)
- Taken together, the most likely diagnosis is pneumonia complicated by hyperglycaemia, dehydration and metabolic acidosis, resulting in confusion and reduced GCS.
- The patient should be started on i.v. fluid (0.9% saline) due to dehydration and low blood pressure, as well as broad spectrum i.v. antibiotics (after taking appropriate cultures) for his chest infection. Oxygen treatment should continue.

Brian's condition quickly deteriorates and his GCS falls to 8/15 (E2, M4, V2). His blood tests show:
FBC Hb 15.7 g/L
WBC 28.3 (neutrophils 25.2) × 10^9/L
Platelets 293 × 10^9/L
U&Es: Na 148 mmol/L
*   K 4.0 mmol/L*
*   Cl 111 mmol/L*
*   Urea 30.1 mmol/L*
*   Creatinine 223 μmol/L*
*   Bicarbonate 15 mmol/L*
*   Glucose 54 mmol/L*

What is the anion gap? What are the potential causes of his acidosis?

Anion gap = (sodium + potassium)
            − (chloride + bicarbonate)

Anion gap = (148 + 4.0) − (111 + 15)
          = 26 (normal 12–20)

His anion gap is high. Causes of high anion gap metabolic acidosis are outlined in Case 1.

What is his calculated plasma osmolarity?

Plasma osmolarity can be calculated from the formula:

2 (sodium + potassium) + urea + glucose

2 (148 + 4.0) + 30 + 54 = 388 (normal 285–295)

His calculated plasma osmolarity is greatly increased.

What does his X-ray show? (Fig. 49)
The X-ray shows right middle lobe pneumonia.

What test would you request next?
- Brian has an infection and metabolic acidosis; therefore, lactic acid levels should be requested. Metformin can also cause lactic acidosis particularly in the presence of renal failure and this is another reason to check lactate levels.

Brian's lactic acid levels are 5.8 mmol/L (1.0–2.4).

What are the diagnoses?
- Chest infection associated with hypoxia and hypotension
- Hyperosmolar non-ketotic hyperglycaemia resulting in dehydration and contributing to low blood pressure
- Metabolic acidosis due to:
  ○ Raised lactic acid (secondary to infection, hypoxia and possibly metformin treatment)
  ○ Deranged renal function may have also contributed to the metabolic acidosis

How would you treat Brian?
Brian requires treatment for:
- Chest infection
- Hyperosmolar non-ketotic hyperglycaemia
  Treatment of the infection and normalization of renal function will correct Brian's metabolic acidosis.

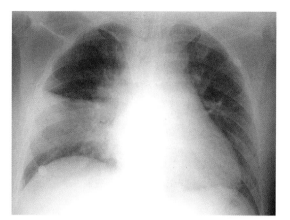

Figure 49 Courtesy of the Radiology Department, University of Leeds.

> **Box 22 Treatment of chest infection**
>
> - Intravenous administration of broad spectrum antibiotics
> - Respiratory support as necessary

What is the prognosis in this case?

- The prognosis of hyperosmolar non-ketotic hypergly-caemia is unfortunately poor
    - More than a third of patients die, commonly from thromboembolic disease

Brian is treated with i.v. antibiotics, fluid and insulin and makes a very good recovery, with all his blood parameters returning to normal 48 h after admission. However, 60 h after his admission, he complains of sudden onset shortness of breath. He denies chest pain.

What is the most likely differential diagnosis?

The most likely differential diagnosis here is:
- Pulmonary embolism
- Relapsed/partially treated chest infection
- Myocardial infarction

What would you do?

- A physical examination, concentrating on the cardiovascular and respiratory system
- ECG
- CXR
- Routine bloods

> **Box 23 Treatment of hyperosmolar non-ketotic hyperglycaemia**
>
> Broadly similar to that of DKA, but with some differences:
> - Fluid: Fluid replacement should be more gentle in hyperosmolar hyperglycaemia compared with DKA as these are older patients and more prone to heart failure with aggressive fluid replacement. In difficult cases, a central line should be inserted that should guide appropriate fluid replacement, to avoid sending the patient into heart failure
> - Insulin: Despite the very high glucose levels in these patients, insulin requirements in non-ketotic hyperosmolar hyperglycaemia are *modest* and, therefore, insulin should be given at 0.5–2 units/h to achieve a gradual drop in blood sugar (around 5 mmol/L/h)
> - Potassium: In uncomplicated hyperosmolar non-ketotic hyperglycaemia, potassium levels do not drop that quickly with treatment due to the absence of acidosis. However, the patient may have acidosis due to other causes (as in the present case) and potassium should, therefore, be monitored carefully
> - Bicarbonate: This is not needed in uncomplicated hyperosmolar hyperglycaemia as the patient is not usually acidotic
> - Precipitating cause(s): Infection is the most common precipitating cause and, therefore, antibiotic cover must be started after appropriate cultures
> - Other measures: Due to high osmolarity and dehydration, thrombotic disease is very common in these patients and, therefore, all should be covered with prophylactic unfractionated heparin (unless haemorrhage is suspected)
> - Monitoring: This should be done regularly with blood samples taken every 2 h in the first 6–8 h to assess response to treatment

On examination, blood pressure is 110/65 (145/85 earlier that day), pulse 104 beats/min regular, O₂ saturation 90% (98% earlier in the day) and respiratory rate 32 breaths/min. Cardiovascular auscultation reveals an additional S3 gallop heart sound. Chest auscultation shows bilateral basal crepitations.

Are these findings compatible with a pulmonary embolus (PE) and why?

- Although PE is a strong possibility, the clinical findings do not fit this diagnosis. In large PE, S3, due to right ventricular dysfunction, may be heard but bilateral basal crepitations are not a feature and these are usually found in left ventricular failure

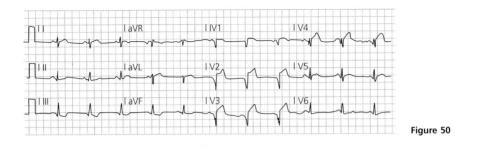

Figure 50

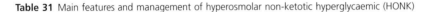

Table 31 Main features and management of hyperosmolar non-ketotic hyperglycaemic (HONK)

Age group affected	Older people with or without a history of diabetes (this could be the first presentation of diabetes)
Glucose	Usually very high (30–80 mmol/L)
Acidosis	Not a feature unless complicated by metabolic acidosis due to other causes (i.e. infection or myocardial infarction)
Serum osmolarity	Very high (>350 mmol)
Ketonuria	There is an absence of severe ketonuria but mild to moderate ketonuria is common (starvation/vomiting)
Precipitating factor	Common: suspect an infection or a vascular event
Management	*Gentle* i.v. fluid
	Gentle i.v. insulin
	Prophylactic heparin is mandatory (unless a bleed is suspected)
	Aggressive use of i.v. antibiotics is encouraged

- The most likely diagnosis here is left ventricular dysfunction resulting in pulmonary oedema

Brian's ECG on admission did not show major abnormalities, his repeat ECG is shown in Fig. 50.

What does the repeat ECG show?
The ECG shows ST elevation in V1-V4 indicating acute anterior-septal myocardial infarction.

What is the diagnosis? How would you explain the absence of chest pain?
- The diagnosis is acute myocardial infarction causing left ventricular dysfunction
- Silent MI (no chest pain) is common in diabetes patients, and this should be taken into account when assessing these individuals

The main features of hyperosmolar non-ketotic hyperglycaemia are summarized in Table 31.

CASE REVIEW

Brian is an older gentleman who is brought into hospital with general deterioration and acute confusion, a common clinical presentation in this age group. The differential diagnosis is wide and includes infection, intoxication with drugs or alcohol, hypoxia, vascular event, intracranial lesion or metabolic/nutritional derangements. An appropriate history, taken usually from relatives or friends, is important to give some clues to the cause of the confusion. Physical examination in this gentleman is consistent with dehydration and chest infection. Subsequent

Continued

tests show biochemical evidence of dehydration with raised glucose, together with hypoxia and lactic acidosis secondary to chest infection. The diagnosis is hyperosmolar non-ketotic hyperglycaemia precipitated by a chest infection. Brian is treated with intravenous antibiotics, fluid and low-dose insulin, subsequently making a good recovery.

However, 2 days later he complains of sudden onset breathlessness without chest pain, which was due to heart failure secondary to silent myocardial infarction. The latter is common in patients with diabetes and should be considered in those with recent history of shortness of breath.

KEY POINTS

- Hyperosmolar non-ketotic hyperglycaemia (HONK) is a rare complication of type 2 diabetes and usually affects the older patient
- HONK carries a poor prognosis as mortality rates can be as high as 50%
- In more than half the cases, HONK occurs in patients who are not known to have diabetes
- HONK is frequently precipitated by an infection or vascular event and patients are severely dehydrated with impaired kidney function and very high plasma glucose levels

- Acidosis is not a feature of HONK, unless it is due to the associated condition, and there is no heavy ketonuria (mild ketonuria may be present due to starvation)
- Patients with HONK should be treated with intravenous:
  - Fluid (careful not to overload and precipitate heart failure)
  - Insulin (only small doses are required)
  - Antibiotics after appropriate cultures (infection is a common precipitating cause)
  - Prophylactic heparin (vascular thrombosis is a common cause of death in patients)

Case 8 — A 42-year-old man with headaches, increased sweating and sexual dysfunction

Adrian, who is 42 years old, is seen by his GP for a 5-month history of headaches, increased sweating, tiredness and sexual dysfunction.

How would you proceed?

Unfortunately, each of the above symptoms is encountered very frequently and at this stage it is unclear whether:

- Symptoms are caused by the same pathology
- Symptoms are the result of a number of independent pathologies

Therefore, more information should be obtained on each of the above symptoms.

- Headache
  - Duration
  - Frequency
  - Location
  - Associated symptoms
  - Provoking and relieving factors
  - Social circumstances (e.g. increased stress at work, family problems)
- Increased sweating
  - Increased sweating and hot flushes can be features of hypogonadism in men
  - Episodes of increased sweating can occur in endocrine diseases such as phaeochromocytoma, acromegaly and carcinoid syndrome
  - May be psychological
  - May be idiopathic
- Tiredness
  - A non-specific symptom, the differential diagnosis of which is discussed elsewhere (Case 10)
- Sexual dysfunction
  - This is discussed in detail elsewhere (Case 21)

Endocrinology and Diabetes: Clinical Cases Uncovered. By R. Ajjan. Published 2009 by Blackwell Publishing, ISBN: 978-1-4051-5726-1

The patient tells you that his:

Headaches are constant, partially relieved by pain killers, generalized but more prominent in the frontal region, have no clear associated symptoms, and he is not suffering increased stress at work or home

Sweating is constant, can be very severe (he sometimes changes his shirt three times/day), and is nocturnal as well as during the day

Sexual dysfunction, he can achieve partial erection but this is insufficient for sexual intercourse, and he has had decreased libido, particularly in the past 3 months

Tiredness is severe, particularly in the past 4 weeks, and is associated with musculoskeletal aches and pains

Adrian says that all the above symptoms started around 5 months ago.

Does the above help in the diagnosis?

The constant headache for 5 months rules out causes of acute and of recurrent headaches.

Box 24 Causes of acute and recurrent headaches

- Acute headache
  - Subarachnoid haemorrhage
  - Meningitis and encephalitis
  - Acute sinusitis (but chronic sinusitis is a possibility)
  - Dental caries
- Recurrent headaches
  - Migraine
  - Cluster headache
  - Trigeminal neuralgia
  - Glaucoma

Subacute headache due to temporal arteritis is unlikely as this occurs after the age of 50 and is commonly associated with scalp tenderness. Therefore, the cause of Adrian's headache is probably related to one of the following diagnoses:

- Tension or psychogenic headache
  - This is a diagnosis of exclusion
- Increased intracranial pressure
  - Usually associated with focal neurological signs
  - Papilloedema on funduscopy
- Pituitary tumours
  - These can cause a headache, which is usually related to tumour size
  - In acromegaly the headache is independent of tumour size

A full neurological examination and funduscopy are both normal. Formal visual field testing is normal.

Would you make a diagnosis of tension headache at this stage?

- A normal neurological examination and the absence of papilloedema on funduscopy make the diagnosis of raised intracranial pressure less likely
- Normal visual field testing does not rule out a pituitary adenoma
- The above information is not enough to make a diagnosis of tension headache
- A more detailed history is required asking specifically for symptoms of pituitary hormone excess

I *Adrian's main symptoms are headache and sweating.*

Which pituitary hormone excess should be ruled out first and what specific questions would you ask?

Increased sweating and headache are common symptoms of patients with acromegaly. Therefore, the questions to be asked should include:

- Changes in glove or shoe size
- Changes in facial appearance
- Arthralgia
- Symptoms of diabetes

Adrian tells you that he has been unable to take off his wedding ring recently and he has had generalized pain in his joints as well as a sensation of pins and needles in his hands.

What signs would you look for?

- Inability to take off the wedding ring and joint pain are consistent with the suspected diagnosis of acromegaly

- The feeling of pins and needles in the hands may be due to carpal tunnel syndrome, which can be associated with acromegaly secondary to soft tissue swelling and compression of the median nerve
- Signs to look for include:
  - Facial appearance (an old photo of the patient is helpful to look for changes): coarse features with prominent supraorbital ridges, increased dental separation, prognathism (protrusion of the lower jaw), enlarged nose, lips and tongue and deep voice
  - Enlarged hands (spade-like hands)
  - Thick, oily skin
  - Hypertension
  - Signs of carpal tunnel syndrome
  - Goitre and organomegalies

Figure 51 (and Fig. 5 in colour plate section) shows a picture of Adrian. He has a deep voice, greasy skin and his blood pressure is 170/95.

How does this help you in making a diagnosis?

- Adrian has prominent supraorbital ridges and coarse facial features
- Deep voice, greasy skin and hypertension are classic features of acromegaly
- Therefore, the patient is very likely to have acromegaly

What biochemical and what radiological tests would you request to confirm the diagnosis?

- Oral glucose tolerance test: in a normal person, plasma growth hormone levels are suppressed after an oral glucose tolerance (OGT) test. In acromegaly there is a failure of growth hormone suppression after OGT
- MRI of the pituitary looking for a pituitary tumour

Adrian fails to suppress plasma growth hormone after OGT and his MRI shows a pituitary tumour measuring 1.5 cm, with no optic nerve compression.

What is the best treatment option for this patient?

- Surgical intervention, usually through a transphenoidal approach, is the preferred treatment
- Radiotherapy is reserved for patients who fail surgical treatment or have contraindication to surgical treatment

Table 32 Main symptoms, signs and complications of growth hormone excess and deficiency.

Growth hormone excess	Growth hormone deficiency
Symptoms	**Symptoms**
Fast growth (in children)	Failure of growth (in children)
Headaches (independent of local tumour effect)	Tiredness
	Depression
Increased sweating	Decreased body mass
Musculoskeletal pains	
Change in glove/ring and shoe size	
Signs	**Signs**
Facial appearance (see text)	Failure of growth and thin skin in children
Soft tissue and skeletal changes	
	No specific signs in adults
Organomegaly	
Visual field defect	
Deficiency of other pituitary hormones	
Complications	**Complications**
Hypertension	Short stature in untreated children
Diabetes	
Colonic polyps and colonic carcinoma	Hypoglycaemia (mainly in children)
Obstructive sleep apnoea	Osteoporosis in adults

What medical treatments are there for patients with acromegaly?

- Somatostatin analogues (octreotide, lanreotide)
- Dopamine agonists (bromocriptine, cabergoline)
- Growth hormone receptor antagonist (pegvisomant)
- Radiotherapy

Box 25 What are the complications of acromegaly?

- Hypertension
- Diabetes or impaired glucose tolerance
- Obstructive sleep apnea
- Increased risk of colonic polyps and colonic carcinoma; therefore, routine colonoscopy is recommended
- Ischaemic heart disease, cerebrovascular disease and heart failure

---

Can clinical and biochemical acromegaly occur in the absence of a primary pituitary pathology?

Yes, very rarely acromegaly may occur secondary to excessive secretion of growth hormone releasing hormone (GHRH)

- Increased secretion from the hypothalamus
- Ectopic secretion from a tumour (such as carcinoid) can result in acromegaly without a primary pituitary pathology but this is rare.

CASE REVIEW

Adrian, a middle-aged man, presents with a few months' history of headaches, increased sweating, tiredness and sexual dysfunction. Further questioning reveals changes in hand size and symptoms compatible with carpal tunnel syndrome. On examination, Adrian has facial features of acromegaly together with greasy skin and hypertension. His neurological examination is normal and he has no visual field defects. An OGT test fails to suppress growth hormone production and a pituitary MRI confirms the presence of an adenoma, indicating that the patient's symptoms are due to a growth hormone secreting pituitary tumour. Treatment of this condition includes surgery and radiotherapy; medical treatment is only partially effective at controlling growth hormone production. Complications of acromegaly include hypertension, diabetes, obstructive sleep apnea, increased risk of colonic carcinoma and vascular disease

KEY POINTS

- Acromegaly is a rare condition that usually results from excessive pituitary growth hormone production. If excessive growth hormone is produced during childhood, it causes gigantism, whereas increased hormone production in adulthood leads to acromegaly
- The main clinical manifestations of acromegaly include:
  - Headaches
  - Increased sweating
  - Tiredness
  - Change in ring, glove or shoe size
  - Typical facial appearances and deep voice
  - Entrapment neuropathies due to soft tissue swelling (carpal tunnel syndrome)
- Surgery is the best treatment option for this condition but radiotherapy and medical treatment are considered for incomplete resection of the tumour, disease relapse or for individuals not fit for surgery
- Complications of acromegaly include:
  - Hypertension
  - Cardiovascular disease
  - Diabetes mellitus
  - Obstructive sleep apnea
  - Increased risk of colonic carcinoma
  - Hypopituitarism and visual field defect

Case 9 Amenorrhoea in an 18-year-old

Sutapa, who is 18, attends her GP clinic complaining of amenorrhoea.

What is the differential diagnosis and how would you proceed with this patient?

Causes of amenorrhoea can be (Fig. 51):

- Physiological
  - Pregnancy: occasionally some patients do not consider this as a possibility, and rarely the physician fails to rule this out initially, ending up requesting complicated, expensive and unnecessary tests
  - Lactation
  - Menopause
- Pathological
  - Primary amenorrhoea: the failure to reach menarche by the age of 16. This may be due to: structural abnormality (such as imperforated hymen, congenital absence of the uterus), genetic disorders (such as Turner's syndrome), testicular feminization syndrome (the individual is genetically a male, with the XY chromosome, but phenotypically a female due to tissue insensitivity to androgens) and causes of secondary amenorrhoea (see below)
  - Secondary amenorrhoea: the cessation of menstrual periods in women who had previously menstruated. Causes can be ovarian [such as polycystic ovary disease, see Case 13, or premature ovarian failure occurring due to chromosomal abnormality (Turner's syndrome), gene mutation in gonadotrophin receptors or autoimmune disease, or iatrogenic premature ovarian failure (chemo- or radiotherapy)], uterine (adhesion in the uterus), pituitary (hypopituitarism or prolactinoma), hypothalamic [excessive exercise (as in professional athletes), severe weight loss, physical or psychological

stress, or hypothalamic tumours or infiltrative lesions] or general endocrine (these are usually associated with menstrual irregularities rather than amenorrhoea and include thyroid dysfunction and Cushing's syndrome)

A full menstrual history is required in order to narrow down the differential diagnosis.

Sutapa tells you that her menarche occurred at the age of 13 and her periods have been regular until 9 months prior to her presentation, when they became less frequent (every 6–7 weeks) and subsequently stopped altogether more than 5 months ago. She had three pregnancy tests (most recent a week ago) and they were all negative.

How does this information help you and what would you do next?

This history of normal menarche and initial regular menses rules out primary causes of amenorrhoea. Pregnancy is ruled out by three negative tests.

At this stage specific questions should be asked targeted at secondary causes of amenorrhoea:

- Ovarian and uterine
  - Hirsutism, obesity (polycystic ovary syndrome)
  - Symptoms of oestrogen deficiency: hot flushes, sweating, mood swings (premature ovarian failure)
  - History of gynaecological procedures or pelvic infections (uterine adhesions)
- Pituitary
  - Symptoms of pituitary failure: growth hormone deficiency, ACTH deficiency (hypoadrenalism) and TSH deficiency (hypothyroidism)
  - Symptoms of prolactin excess: galactorrhoea (breast milk production)
- Hypothalamic
  - History of excessive exercise
  - History of recent stress
  - History of weight loss

Endocrinology and Diabetes: Clinical Cases Uncovered. By R. Ajjan.
Published 2009 by Blackwell Publishing, ISBN: 978-1-4051-5726-1

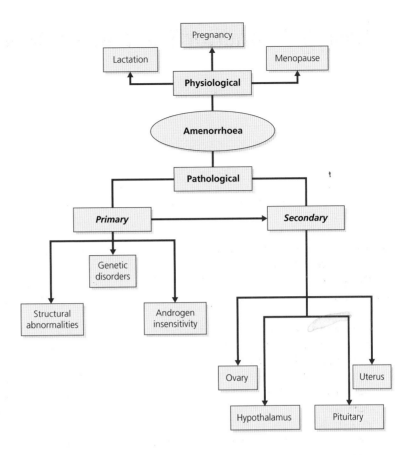

Figure 51 Causes of amenorrhoea.

Sutapa denies any change in lifestyle or weight, and she is not having any major stress in her life. However, she mentions galactorrhoea that is becoming an embarrassing problem.

What signs would you look for?

• Galactorrhoea: this can be confirmed on physical examination
• Visual field defects: abnormalities suggest a large pituitary tumour
• Rule out clinical pituitary insufficiency (see Case 4)

Sutapa has normal visual fields and no signs to suggest pituitary failure. Galactorrhoea is confirmed on physical examination.

What is the most likely diagnosis and how would you confirm this?

• The most likely diagnosis is a prolactinoma (Table 33)

Table 33 Presentation of prolactinomas.

Symptoms related to excess prolactin	Symptoms related to the mass effect
Galactorrhoea (90% of women, 10% of men)	Headaches
Menstrual disturbances in the majority	Visual field defects
Reduced libido in both women and men	Hypopituitarism
Erectile dysfunction in men	Cranial nerve palsies (invasion of the cavernous sinus or pituitary apoplexy)

• Diagnosis can be confirmed by measuring plasma prolactin levels

I *Plasma prolactin is 14600 mU/L (normal range <600 mU/L).*

Does this confirm the diagnosis?

Yes, this confirms the diagnosis of a prolactinoma. Difficulties can arise when prolactin levels are less than 6000 mU/L, which may be due to a prolactinoma but may equally be due to a large pituitary tumour with a "stalk effect", consequently resulting in raised prolactin levels.

What is the differential diagnosis of raised plasma prolactin?

- Physiological
  - Pregnancy
  - Nipple stimulation
  - Sexual intercourse
  - Stress (taking a blood sample from some individuals can be a stressful experience and may result in modest elevation of plasma prolactin)
- Drug treatment, there is an extensive list of drugs that can result in raised prolactin including:
  - Dopamine receptor antagonists (metoclopramide)
  - Neuroleptics (such as chlorpromazine, haloperidol)
  - Antidepressants
  - Opiates
  - Antiretroviral treatment
- Endocrine causes
  - Hypothyroidism (raised TRH stimulates prolactin secretion)
- Metabolic
  - Renal failure (decreased excretion of prolactin)
- Hypothalamic
  - Mass compressing the stalk
  - Infiltrative disease
- Pituitary
  - Prolactinoma
  - Large pituitary tumour causing stalk compression

MRI of the pituitary shows a large pituitary adenoma measuring 1.8 cm in diameter with no optic nerve compression.

What is the best treatment option?

- Dopamine agonists (bromocriptine and cabergoline) do not only reduce plasma prolactin levels but also result in shrinkage of prolactinomas
- Surgery is usually the best treatment for most pituitary tumours *except* for prolactinomas, where medical treatment is first line and surgery is reserved for non-responders to dopamine agonists
- Successful treatment is associated with a drop in prolactin levels, reduction in tumour size and normalization of menstrual cycles

---

Box 26 Difference between micro- and macroprolactinomas

- Microprolactinomas are tumours measuring ≤1 cm in diameter
- Macroprolactinomas are tumours measuring >1 cm in diameter

- Patients started on dopamine agonists should be counselled regarding pregnancy

Sutapa comes to see you 8 months after starting cabergoline treatment to tell you that she is now pregnant.

What would you do with her treatment?

- In patients with microprolactinomas, it is usually safe to stop the treatment as tumour expansion is very rare
- In patients with macroadenomas, management remains controversial and should be individualized. A large number of patients continue on dopamine agonists, which, particularly bromocriptine, seem to be safe in pregnancy
- This patient should be referred to an endocrinologist with experience in managing pituitary pathologies

Symptoms and signs of pituitary prolactinoma are summarized in Table 33.

CASE REVIEW

Sutapa is a young woman who presents with secondary amenorrhoea and galactorrhoea. Pregnancy is ruled out as the cause of her amenorrhoea, an important step in investigating amenorrhoea in order to avoid unnecessary investigations. Apart from galactorrhoea, her physical examination is unremarkable and she does not have signs of pituitary hormone deficiency. Subsequent tests confirm raised plasma prolactin levels, an abnormality that can be due to a large number of reasons including physiological causes, certain medications, endocrine and metabolic conditions. Further investigations confirm a pituitary macroadenoma as the cause of her raised prolactin. Treatment of prolactinomas is usually medical and surgery is rarely required.

KEY POINTS

- Secondary amenorrhoea is a common condition and pregnancy should always be ruled out as a cause before embarking on expensive investigations
- Causes of secondary amenorrhoea include abnormalities in:
  - Hypothalamus (increased stress)
  - Pituitary (pituitary tumours in general, prolactinomas in particular)
  - Ovary (polycystic ovary disease)
  - Uterus (uterine adhesions following infections)
- In addition to menstrual irregularities, raised prolactin may cause galactorrhoea
- There is an extensive list for the causes of hyperprolactinaemia, including:
  - Physiological (pregnancy, sexual intercourse, nipple stimulation, stress)
  - Pituitary tumours (prolactinomas or other tumours with stalk compression)
  - Drugs (metoclopramide, antipsychotics and antidepressants, opiates, HIV treatment)
  - Metabolic and endocrine (hypothyroidism, polycystic ovary syndrome, chronic renal failure)
- Treatment of hyperprolactinaemia should be directed at the cause. In the case of a pituitary prolactinoma, the treatment is usually medical, and not surgical, using dopamine agonists (bromocriptine, cabergoline)

PART 2: CASES

Case 10 A 28-year-old with tiredness and abnormal thyroid function postpartum

One week after her 28th birthday and 6 weeks after giving birth, Nicola consults her GP, with a 3–4-week history of extreme tiredness. Her GP checks her TFTs and results show: FT4 5.1 pmol/L (normal range 10.0–25.0 pmol/L) TSH 2.1 mIU/L (normal range 0.2–6.0 mIU/L)

What questions would you ask?

Results show a low FT4 with inappropriately "normal" TSH, indicating secondary hypothyroidism. Questions should be directed towards symptoms of pituitary failure:

• Tiredness (hypothyroidism, hypoadrenalism and growth hormone deficiency)
• Gastrointestinal symptoms, weight loss (hypoadrenalism)
• Dizziness due to low blood pressure (hypoadrenalism)
• Failure of lactation (prolactin deficiency)

Nicola tells you that she managed to breast feed for only a week post delivery. She has had dizziness for at least 3 weeks and has been feeling very weak with reduced appetite and rapid weight loss.

What signs would you look for?

• Dizziness, weakness, reduced appetite and failure to lactate are strongly suggestive of pituitary failure
• The following should be assessed in individuals with suspected pituitary failure:
  ○ Blood pressure: low blood pressure is seen in ACTH deficiency but it can be in the normal range in patients with pituitary failure due to preserved aldosterone production by the adrenal gland (which is mainly controlled by the renin-angiotensin system)

  ○ Thyroid status: looking for signs of hypothyroidism
  ○ Visual field: pituitary failure may occur in the presence of a large pituitary adenoma

What investigations would you request?

Investigation of pituitary insufficiency involves (Fig. 52):
• Hormonal tests
  ○ Basal hormone levels: 9:00 am cortisol, very low levels can confirm hypoadrenalism (primary or secondary). However, levels in the low-normal range are non-diagnostic and dynamic tests are required (see below); prolactin, during the period of breast feeding, prolactin levels are high and low levels early in the postpartum period are suggestive of hypopituitarism; sex hormones [oestrogen (in females), testosterone (in males), FSH and LH] are usually requested in individuals with suspected pituitary failure. However, sex hormone levels can be difficult to interpret shortly after giving birth
  ○ Dynamic tests: glucagon stimulation test (GST), insulin stress test (IST), low-dose synacthen test (LDST)

  GST and IST assess cortisol and growth hormone reserve, whereas LDST determines cortisol reserve only (Fig. 52)
• Imaging
  ○ MRI of the pituitary gland

Nicola's blood tests show low prolactin with inadequate cortisol and growth hormone response to IST.

What is your diagnosis?

• Abnormal IST, low prolactin and low FT4 with normal TSH is diagnostic of pituitary failure
• Remember that in early pituitary failure an individual may only have one or two hormonal deficiencies, and as the condition progresses lack of other hormones becomes evident

---

Endocrinology and Diabetes: Clinical Cases Uncovered. By R. Ajjan. Published 2009 by Blackwell Publishing, ISBN: 978-1-4051-5726-1

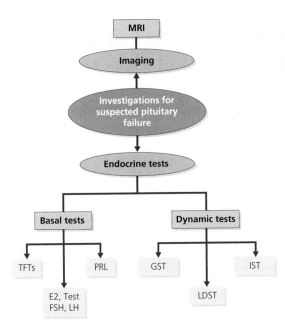

Figure 52 Investigations for suspected pituitary failure. E2, oestradiol; FSH, follicle stimulating hormone; GST, glucagon stimulation test; IST, insulin stress test; LDST, low-dose synacthen test; LH, luteinizing hormone; MRI, magnetic resonance imaging; PRL, prolactin; Test, testosterone; TFTs, thyroid function tests.

Nicola tells you that she had a difficult labour and lost large amounts of blood.

What is the most likely aetiology of her pituitary failure and what is the differential diagnosis?

- Severe blood loss can cause infarction in the pituitary gland secondary to hypotension, resulting in hypopituitarism and is called Sheehan's syndrome. Fortunately, improved obstetric care in the developed world has made this a rare complication
- The differential diagnosis for the causes of hypopituitarism include:
  - ○ Tumours affecting the pituitary gland
  - ○ Radiotherapy of the head
  - ○ Pituitary apoplexy
  - ○ Infiltrative disease (sarcoidosis, haemachromatosis)
  - ○ Pituitary infection (abscess of the pituitary gland)
  - ○ Head trauma

How would you manage this patient?

- An MRI of the pituitary should be requested to rule out other causes of pituitary pathology
- She will need hormonal replacements to cover her multiple hormone deficiencies

Which hormone should be replaced first?

- Cortisol should be the first hormone to get replaced. If thyroxine is given before adequate cortisol replacement it may precipitate a hypoadrenal crisis. Therefore, in panhypopituitarism, cortisol is replaced first followed 48 h later by thyroid hormone replacement
- Female hormones should be replaced using an adequate combination of oestrogen and progesterone
- In men with hypopituitarism, testosterone should be replaced
- Certain criteria are needed to replace growth hormone and this is best left to an expert in this field

CASE REVIEW

Six weeks after giving birth, Nicola seeks medical advice for 3–4 weeks' history of extreme tiredness. An initial blood test shows low FT4 with inappropriately normal TSH, indicating a diagnosis of secondary hypothyroidism. Specific questioning directed at pituitary hormone deficiency strongly suggests pituitary failure manifested as inability to breast feed (absence of prolactin) and symptoms consistent with steroid hormone deficiency (absence of ACTH). Further investigations confirm the deficiency of several pituitary hormones and a diagnosis of pituitary failure is made. In patients with pituitary failure MRI imaging is essential to rule out a pituitary pathology. Severe blood loss during delivery may cause pituitary failure through infarction, known as Sheehan's syndrome, which is a possible diagnosis in this case. In individuals with multiple pituitary hormone deficiency, cortisol should be replaced first, as early replacement with thyroxine may precipitate an adrenal crisis. Cortisol replacement is important in any individual with suspected adrenal or pituitary failure, with the treatment started even before initiating investigations in case the patient is acutely unwell.

KEY POINTS

- Low thyroid hormones with inappropriately low or normal TSH should raise the suspicion of secondary hypothyroidism
- Individuals with secondary hypothyroidism should be investigated for other pituitary hormone deficiency using static and stimulatory hormonal tests
- Clinical features of hypopituitarism include:
  - Growth arrest in children and tiredness in adults (GH deficiency)
  - Amenorrhoea in women (FSH and LH deficiency) and erectile dysfunction in men (LH deficiency)
  - Weight loss and tiredness (ACTH deficiency)
  - Symptoms of hypothyroidism (TSH deficiency)
  - Failure of lactation (prolactin deficiency)
  - Polyuria and polydipsia (ADH deficiency): only occurs if the posterior pituitary is involved in the pathological process
- Individuals with pituitary failure should be investigated for the aetiology of the condition, including:
  - Pituitary or parapituitary tumours
  - Pituitary infarction
  - Infiltrative disease (histiocytosis, haemachromatosis, sarcoidosis)
  - Previous radiotherapy
  - Trauma (following head injury)
- Management of pituitary failure requires replacement of the deficient hormone(s) and treatment of the cause

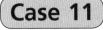

Case 11 A 33-year-old man with polyuria and polydipsia

Peter, aged 33, is referred by his GP following a 2-month history of polyuria and polydipsia. The patient says that the problem got worse recently and he can pass up to 6 L of urine per day.

What is the differential diagnosis at this stage?

The differential diagnosis of polyuria and polydipsia includes:

- Diabetes (type 1 or type 2)
- Hypercalcaemia
- Chronic renal failure
- Diabetes insipidus
- Diuretic abuse
- Psychogenic

It is important to note that some patients complain of polyuria without an actual increase in their urine output and urine volumes should be measured over 24 h to confirm the diagnosis of polyuria in uncertain cases.

What symptoms and signs would you be looking for to narrow down the differential diagnosis?

- Diabetes
  - Skin infections
  - Blurred vision
  - Overweight (T2DM)
  - History of weight loss (T1DM)
  - Tiredness
- Hypercalcaemia
  - Anorexia
  - Vomiting
  - Abdominal pain
  - Constipation
  - Lethargy
  - Confusion
  - Depression
- Chronic renal failure
  - Previous history of renal injury
  - Anorexia
  - Lethargy
  - Itching
  - Anaemia
  - Oedema
  - Hypertension
- Diabetes insipidus (DI)
  - History of head injury
  - Intracranial tumours
  - Chronic inflammatory conditions (tuberculosis, histiocytosis, sarcoidosis)
  - Use of drugs (lithium, demeclocycline)

What tests would you request at this stage?

- Plasma glucose
- Plasma calcium
- U&Es
- Plasma and urine osmolarities

Blood tests show:

Fasting glucose	5.1 mmol/L
Corrected calcium	2.35 mmol/L
Sodium	147 mmol/L
Potassium	3.9 mmol/L
Urea	5.5 mmol/L
Creatinine	88 µmol/L
Plasma osmolarity	300 mOsm/kg
Urine osmolarity	155 mOsm/kg

What do these results indicate?

The above results rule out the following as the cause of this patient's symptoms:

Endocrinology and Diabetes: Clinical Cases Uncovered. By R. Ajjan. Published 2009 by Blackwell Publishing, ISBN: 978-1-4051-5726-1

PART 2: CASES

Table 34 Results of water deprivation test.

Time	Plasma osmolarity	Urine osmolarity
0 h	300	158
4 h	306	154
5 h (i.m. vasopressin given)	308	155
8 h	295	835

- Diabetes
- Hypercalcaemia
- Chronic renal failure

The high plasma sodium and increased plasma osmolarity with inappropriately low urine osmolarity suggest a diagnosis of diabetes insipidus.

What test would you request to confirm the diagnosis?

A water deprivation test with desmopressin administration.

The results of Peter's water deprivation test are shown in Table 34.

How would you interpret these results?

- These results confirm DI, as the patient fails to concentrate his urine despite increasing plasma osmolarity
- Concentration of urine after vasopressin administration, together with a fall in plasma osmolarity, is consistent with a diagnosis of cranial DI (lack of ADH)

The patient had an X-ray done a week ago (Fig. 53a) due to persistent cough. He is also complaining of painful and red skin eruptions on his shins, which he has had for 3 days (Fig. 53b, colour plate section).

What abnormality can you see on the CXR? What is the skin lesion? Can you give a unifying diagnosis?

The CXR (Fig. 53a) shows bilateral hilar enlargement. Hilar lymphadenopathy can be seen in:
- Sarcoidosis
- Infection (tuberculosis)
- Malignancy (lymphoma)

The red and painful skin lesions are characteristic of erythema nodosum, which can be seen in:

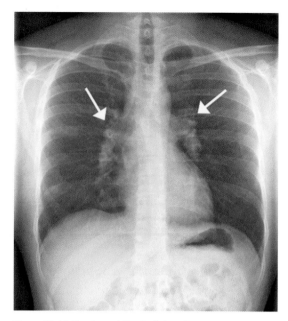

Figure 53 (a) Courtesy of the Radiology Department, University of Leeds.

- Infections
  - Bacterial (*Streptococcus*, tuberculosis)
  - Viral
  - Fungal
- Inflammatory bowel disease
  - Malignancy
  - Sarcoidosis
  - Drugs (oral contraceptives, sulphonamides, penicillin)

Taken together, the most likely unifying diagnosis is sarcoidosis causing DI, secondary to the inflammatory infiltrate in the posterior pituitary. Another remote possibility is tuberculosis.

What imaging would you request in this patient?

MRI of the pituitary.

What is the treatment of cranial DI?

- Treat the cause
- Desmopressin can be given:
  - Orally
  - Intranasally
  - Injections

Box 27 Causes of diabetes insipidus

These can be divided into:
- Cranial
  - Familial
  - Acquired: head injury, pituitary tumours, infiltrative disease (tuberculosis, sarcoidosis, histiocytosis), infections (meningitis or encephalitis), vascular events, idiopathic (no cause found)
- Nephrogenic
  - Familial
  - Acquired: drugs (lithium, demeclocycline), electrolyte abnormalities (hypokalaemia, hypercalcaemia), chronic renal disease

---

What is the treatment of nephrogenic DI?

- Treat the cause and maintain adequate fluid intake

- Drug treatment (only partially effective) includes:
  - Thiazide diuretics
  - Prostaglandin synthase inhibitors such as indomethacin

What is the main difference in serum and urine osmolarities comparing DI with psychogenic polydipsia?

- In both DI and psychogenic polydipsia the urine osmolarity is low
- Plasma osmolarity is high in DI but low or low-normal in psychogenic polydipsia
- In difficult cases, a water deprivation test should be performed to differentiate between these two conditions

Table 35 summarizes the main features of cranial and nephrogenic DI as well as psychogenic polydipsia.

Table 35 Main features of cranial and nephrogenic DI and psychogenic polydipsia.

	Cranial DI	Nephrogenic DI	Psychogenic polydipsia
Posmo	High-normal or high	High-normal or high	Low-normal or low
Uosmo	Low	Low	Low
After water deprivation test			
Posmo	High	High	Normal
Uosmo	Low	Low	Normal
After desmopressin administration			
Posmo	Normal	High	Normal
Uosmo	Increase (normalizes)	Low	Normal

Posmo, plasma osmolarity; uosmo, urine osmolarity.

CASE REVIEW

Peter consults his doctor with a 2-month history of polyuria and polydipsia. Diuretic abuse, diabetes, hypercalcaemia and chronic renal failure are ruled out as a cause for his symptoms. Diabetes insipidus is suspected, which is confirmed following a water deprivation test. An improvement in urine osmolarity after vasopressin injection indicates a diagnosis of cranial DI (deficiency of ADH), rather than nephrogenic DI (reduced responsiveness of the kidneys to ADH). The patient has an abnormal CXR with bilateral hilar enlargement and a skin lesion consistent with erythema nodosum. This strongly suggests a diagnosis of sarcoidosis as a cause for this patient's DI. Treatment of cranial DI is replacement with desmopressin, which can be given orally, intranasally or subcutaneously.

KEY POINTS

- Diabetes insipidus is a known cause of passing large amounts of diluted urine. It should be differentiated from other causes of polyuria, including:
  - Diabetes
  - Hypercalcaemia
  - Psychogenic polydipsia
- Causes of DI include:
  - Cranial: infiltrative disease (histiocytosis, haemachromatosis, sarcoidosis), pituitary or parapituitary tumours, pituitary infarction, trauma (following head injury), or rare familial disorders
  - Nephrogenic: drugs (lithium, demeclocycline), chronic renal disease, electrolyte imbalance (hypercalcaemia, hypokalaemia), or familial disorders
- Investigations for DI include:
  - Water deprivation test
  - Pituitary imaging
- Treatment includes:
  - Desmopressin with adequate fluid intake
  - Treat the cause

A 62-year-old man with tiredness and hyponatraemia

Max, a 62-year-old gentleman, is seen by his GP with a few days' history of severe tiredness. Routine blood tests are requested and these show:

Na+	119 mmol/L
K+	3.4 mmol/L
Urea	4.2 mmol/L
Creatinine	65 μmol/L.

What differential diagnosis would you think of at this stage?

Hyponatraemia is a common finding and not infrequently mismanaged. A large proportion of patients with hyponatraemia are initially diagnosed as syndrome of inappropriate ADH secretion (SIADH) without proper assessment. Hyponatraemia may be due to (Fig. 54):
- Sodium loss and dehydration (in which case the patient is hypovolaemic):
  - Use of diuretics (a very common cause)
  - Diarrhoea
  - Vomiting
  - Renal disease and salt wasting
  - Mineralocorticoid deficiency: hypoaldosteronism or Addison's disease
- Water excess with euvolaemia:
  - SIADH
  - Glucocorticoid deficiency
  - Hypothyroidism
- Water excess with hypervolaemia:
  - Cirrhosis
  - Cardiac failure
  - Nephrotic syndrome

What would you like to do at this stage?

- A full medical history, including a review of current medications
- Clinical examination

Max tells you that he started to feel increasingly tired 6 weeks ago, lost his appetite and this was associated with weight loss. Past medical history includes temporal lobe epilepsy for which he has been on treatment for more than 15 years. On examination he looks well hydrated and his physical examination is unremarkable.

How would the above information help in establishing a diagnosis?

- Max is clinically well hydrated
- The urea is not elevated further suggesting that the patient is well hydrated
  - It should be noted that in malnourished individuals (such as alcoholics) urea can be very low, and, therefore, urea in the normal range does not rule out dehydration
- Taken together, hyponatraemia secondary to dehydration is unlikely here
- A normal physical examination further rules out:
  - Cirrhosis
  - Cardiac failure
  - Nephrotic syndrome
  - Hypothyroidism (but in some case individuals with hypothyroidism may have very few clinical signs)

What is the likely diagnosis from the clinical evidence given above?

- The likely diagnosis is SIADH
- Glucocorticoid deficiency and hypothyroidism remain two possibilities and these should be ruled out

What tests would you request to confirm the diagnosis?

- Plasma osmolarity
- Urine osmolarity with urinary electrolytes
- TFTs (to rule out the possibility of hypothyroidism)
- A random cortisol with or without a synacthen test (to rule out glucocorticoid deficiency)

Endocrinology and Diabetes: Clinical Cases Uncovered. By R. Ajjan. Published 2009 by Blackwell Publishing, ISBN: 978-1-4051-5726-1

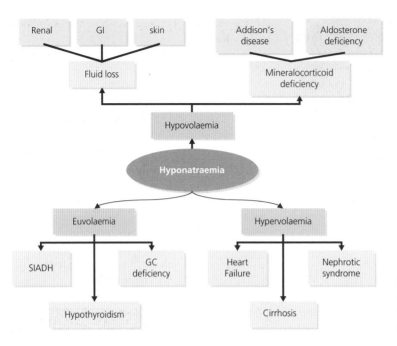

Figure 54 Causes of hyponatraemia. GC, glucocorticoid; SIADH, syndrome of inappropriate antidiuretic hormone secretion.

Before the blood is taken for the above tests, what would you like to know?

A review of current medications is essential (particularly the use of diuretics and thyroxine).

> The list of medications includes carbamazepine and paracetamol as required.
> Max's tests showed:
> Plasma osmolarity   243 mOsm
> Urine osmolarity   487 mOsm
> Urine sodium   52 mmol/L
> Random cortisol   620 nmol/L
> FT4   21 pmol/L
> TSH   1.8 mIU/L.

What is the diagnosis?

- Max has a normal thyroid function and no evidence of glucocorticoid deficiency
- Max has:
  - Low plasma osmolarity
  - Inappropriately high urine osmolarity
  - High urinary sodium excretion
  The diagnosis is, therefore, SIADH.

What is the aetiology of SIADH in this case?

- A possibility is carbamazepine use

- A previous U&Es result would help in differentiating hyponatraemia due to drug use

> Max had his U&Es checked 6 months ago which showed:
> Sodium   136 mmol/L
> Potassium   4.3 mmol/L
> Urea   3.8 mmol/L
> Creatinine   67 µmol/L.

Box 28 Causes of SIADH

- Malignancy
- Chest infections (particularly atypical pneumonia)
- Abnormalities in the central nervous system
  - Infections
  - Head injuries
  - Vascular disorders
- Metabolic
  - Porphyria
- Drugs
  - Chemotherapy
  - Psychiatric drugs
  - Anti-epileptics (carbamazepine)
  - Antidiabetics (chlorpropamide)
- Idiopathic

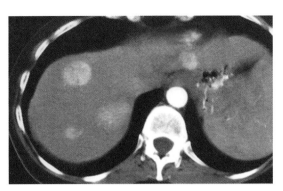

Figure 55 Courtesy of the Radiology Department, University of Leeds.

What do these results indicate?

The normal sodium 6 months earlier makes SIADH secondary to carbamazepine use unlikely.

What would you do now?

• Malignancy as a cause of SIADH should be ruled out, particularly in view of the recent history of weight loss
• A number of tests can be requested at this stage including:
  ○ CXR
  ○ Abdominal ultrasound
  ○ Prostate specific antigen (PSA; rule out cancer of the prostate)

• If the above tests are negative, whole body CT should be considered
   The patient's abdominal ultrasound is shown in Fig. 55.

What does this section of the liver show? What is the likely diagnosis?

The ultrasound shows multiple hepatic metastases, and, therefore, the likely cause of SIADH is metastatic malignancy.

How would you manage Max's hyponatraemia?

• Fluid restriction (750–1500 mL/day)
• Treat the underlying cause if possible
• In long-term cases, demeclocycline can be tried (which induces nephrogenic diabetes insipidus)

> **!RED FLAG**
>
> Hyponatraemia should be corrected slowly (0.5 mmol/h and less than 10 mmol/24 h) to avoid the rare complication of central pontine myelinolysis.
>
> In severe hyponatraemia with neurological signs (seizures), rapid correction of the low sodium to a 'safe level' may be necessary and can be achieved by infusion of hypertonic saline.

PART 2: CASES

CASE REVIEW

Max, who is 62 years old, consults his doctor with a history of tiredness. Initial investigations show significant hyponatraemia and he is, therefore, admitted to hospital for further management. Hyponatraemia can occur in the presence of hypovolaemia, euvolaemia or hypervolaemia. Assessing hydration status of the patient is important to plan appropriate investigations. Max appears well hydrated and on further questioning it became apparent that he lost significant weight recently due to poor appetite. His clinical presentation, plasma and urine osmolarities and urinary electrolytes are consistent with SIADH. The possibility of drug-induced SIADH is considered as

Max is on long-term treatment with carbamazepine. However, his plasma sodium levels 6 months earlier, when he was on the same treatment, were normal casting doubts about this diagnosis. He is subsequently investigated for the possibility of malignancy as a cause of his SIADH and liver ultrasound confirms the presence of multiple metastases. Max is subsequently managed by fluid restriction and treatment of the underlying pathology is considered. Correction of hyponatraemia should be done gradually, particularly if sodium levels are very low, to avoid the rare but serious complication of central pontine myelinolysis.

KEY POINTS

- Hyponatraemia is a common condition in hospitalized patients
- It is very important to assess fluid status in individuals with hyponatraemia (hypovolaemic, euvolaemic, hypervolaemic) together with a review of their medications (diuretics and inappropriate fluid replacement probably remain the commonest cause of hyponatraemia in hospitalized patients)
- Causes of hyponatraemia include:
  - With hypovolaemia: renal salt loss (diuretics, tubular defect, mineralocorticoid deficiency) and gastrointestinal loss (vomiting, diarrhoea)
  - With euvolaemia: SIADH, glucocorticoid deficiency and hypothyroidism
  - With hypervolaemia: cirrhosis, heart failure and renal failure
- Diagnosis of SIADH is confirmed by demonstrating low plasma osmolarity in the presence of high urine osmolarity and high urinary electrolyte concentration
- Treatment of SIADH includes:
  - Treat the cause
  - Fluid restriction
  - Medical treatment is considered in difficult cases
- Treatment of other causes of hyponatraemia should be directed at the cause

Case 13 Excess hair in a 29-year-old woman

Julie is 29 years old and is complaining of excess hair on her neck, chin and body.

What differential diagnosis would you consider at this stage?

Excess hair or hirsutism is a common complaint affecting more than 10% of women.

Causes include:
- Polycystic ovary syndrome (PCOS): common
- Familial or racial (for example Mediterranean origin): common
- Drugs (phenytoin, corticosteroids, cyclosporine, anabolic steroids, minoxidil)
- Congenital adrenal hyperplasia: rare
- Cushing's syndrome: rare
- Ovarian and adrenal tumours: rare
- Idiopathic

What questions would you ask to try to establish a diagnosis?

- Onset: long history or recent problem; a recent history of hirsutism, particularly in severe disease, warrants prompt and full investigations
- Family history of hirsutism (familial hirsutism)
- Menstrual history: normal periods effectively rule out significant hyperandrogenism (ovarian and adrenal tumours unlikely)
- History of virilism
  - Change of voice
  - Clitoromegaly
  - Frontal bolding
  - Increased muscle mass
- Distinguish between:
  - Androgen-dependent hair growth: coarse and pig-

mented hair occurring in areas where men normally develop hair growth
  - Androgen-independent hair growth: excess vellus hair over face and trunk

What signs would you be looking for?

- Assess severity and distribution of hirsutism (special tables can be used for this)
- Distinguish between androgen-dependent and androgen-independent hair growth
- Look for signs of virilization: these are usually associated with an androgen-producing tumour
- Abdominal examination: looking for abdominal masses (ovarian tumour)
- Signs of Cushing's syndrome
- Acanthosis nigricans: this can be associated with insulin resistance suggesting a diagnosis of PCOS

Julie tells you she always had excess body hair but this started to worsen in the past 18 months or so. Her periods have been irregular for the past 8 years occurring every 2–3 months. There is a family history of T2DM but there is no history of hirsutism.

On examination, she is overweight with a BMI of 32.4 kg/m². She has a lesion in her axilla, shown in Fig. 56 (colour plate section). She has excess hair on her chest, chin, abdomen and inner thighs (noted as "mild"). There are no signs of virilization.

Given the information above, what is the most likely diagnosis?

The most likely diagnosis is PCOS supported by:
- Long history of hirsutism and oligomenorrhoea
- Obesity
- Excessive hair in androgenic distribution
- Absence of signs of virilization
- Presence of acanthosis nigricans suggesting increased insulin resistance, which is a feature of PCOS

Endocrinology and Diabetes: Clinical Cases Uncovered. By R. Ajjan. Published 2009 by Blackwell Publishing, ISBN: 978-1-4051-5726-1

Can you rule out an androgen secreting tumour from history and examination?

An androgen secreting tumour in this patient is highly unlikely due to:

- Slow onset of symptoms
- Absence of virilization

What tests would you request to confirm the diagnosis?

- Testosterone: normal or mildly elevated in PCOS (<5 nmol/L)
- SHBG low in more than half of PCOS women, consequently resulting in high free androgens
- FSH and LH: high LH/FSH ratio in two-thirds of PCOS
- Ovarian ultrasound: typical ovarian morphology can be seen in the majority of PCOS patients (particularly using transvaginal ultrasound)
- Other tests:
  - Fasting glucose (diabetes in 10% and impaired glucose tolerance in 40% of PCOS patients)
  - Lipids

Julie's blood tests show the following (normal ranges):
Testosterone 2.8 nmol/L (1–2.5)
SHBG 9 nmol/L (22–120)
FSH 2.4 U/L
LH 5.3 U/L
Fasting glucose 6.8 mmol/L
Triglyceride 2.1 mmol/L
Cholesterol 4.8 mmol/L
Prolactin 445 (<600 mU/L)
17-OH progesterone 12 nmol/L (1–20)
Abdominal ultrasound: Normal appearance of the ovaries

Why did Julie have her prolactin and 17-OH progesterone checked?

- Prolactin was checked as a routine test investigating her irregular periods (see Cases 4 & 10)
- 17-OH progesterone was checked to rule out the possibility of congenital adrenal hyperplasia (discussed in Case 13)

What is the diagnosis?

Julie has:

- Mildly elevated testosterone
- Low SHBG (consequently increasing the levels of unbound/free testosterone)

- Raised LH/FSH ratio
- Impaired fasting glucose

Taken together, the most likely diagnosis is PCOS. The failure to detect polycystic ovaries on abdominal ultrasound does not rule out the diagnosis, particularly as this has a lower sensitivity compared with transvaginal ultrasound.

What other blood test(s) would you request?

This patient should undergo a glucose tolerance test due to her impaired fasting glucose.

What are the treatment options for Julie?

- Weight loss, this is important as it results in:
  - Reduction in hyperandrogenism
  - Increase in insulin sensitivity

  A minor reduction of weight by 5% can result in 50% improvement in hirsutism.
- Oral contraceptive pills (OCP), the most commonly used is Dianette which contains:
  - Oestrogen (ethinyl oestradiol)
  - Androgen receptor blocker (cyproterone acetate)
- Insulin sensitizers
  - Metformin: has been successfully used to restore ovulation and induce fertility in PCOS
  - Thiazolidinediones: rosiglitazone and pioglitazone are less frequently used compared with metformin
- Anti-androgen treatment
  - Cyproterone acetate: increases hepatic androgen clearance
  - Spironolactone: weak anti-androgen
  - Flutamide: strong anti-androgen
- 5α-reductase inhibitors
  - Finasteride: inhibits the conversion of testosterone to the potent androgen dihydrotestosterone

  It should be noted that women with PCOS receiving pharmacological treatment should be given appropriate contraceptive advice.

Julie is very keen on starting a family.

What advice would you give her and would you start her on any pharmacological treatment?

- The importance of weight loss should be emphasized
- Metformin treatment has been shown to restore ovulation in some patients with PCOS and therapy with this agent is a possibility. Other treatment options are summarized in Table 19, p. 41.

CASE REVIEW

Julie is a young woman who presents with hirsutism and menstrual irregularities. More than 10% of women have varying degrees of hirsutism, with the commonest causes being polycystic ovary syndrome and familial or racial predisposition. It is important to take a full history including onset of symptoms, menstrual history and markers of virilism. Severity of the condition should be assessed and causes of secondary hirsutism should be looked for. Julie is overweight and is found to have acanthosis nigricans, a condition associated with insulin resistance, together with excess hair in androgenic distribution with no signs of virilism. The most likely diagnosis is polycystic ovary syndrome, which is further supported by biochemical tests showing mildly raised testosterone with low SHBG and elevated LH/FSH ratio together with impaired fasting glucose. Treatment for this condition includes weight reduction, oral contraceptive pills, insulin sensitizers and anti-androgen treatment.

KEY POINTS

- Hirsutism in women is a common complaint
- Causes of hirsutism include:
  - Common: polycystic ovary syndrome (PCOS), and familial or racial
  - Rare: adrenal or ovarian tumours, congenital adrenal hyperplasia and Cushing's syndrome
- Rapid onset of symptoms, particularly in the presence of virilization, warrants prompt and full investigations
- The majority of women with hirsutism have PCOS, which is further characterized by:
  - Menstrual irregularities
  - Obesity
  - Insulin resistance (hyperinsulinaemia with or without high glucose levels)
- PCOS is diagnosed by:
  - Clinical presentation
  - Low sex hormone binding globulin (SHBG) with or without mildly elevated testosterone levels
  - Raised LH/FSH ratio
  - Cystic ovaries on ultrasound (transvaginal is more accurate than transabdominal)
- Treatment of PCOS includes:
  - Weight loss
  - Oral contraceptive pills (result in elevated SHBG and, hence, lower free testosterone)
  - Insulin sensitizers (metformin is the most commonly used agent)
  - Androgen receptor blockers (cyproterone acetate, spironolactone)
  - 5α-reductase inhibitors (finasteride)

Case 14 A 52-year-old woman with paroxysmal atrial fibrillation and abnormal thyroid function

Bridget, who is 52 years old with a past medical history of paroxysmal atrial fibrillation, was referred with the following thyroid function results:

FT4   30.1 pmol/L (10.0–25.0)

FT3   4.7 pmol/L (3.4–7.2)

TSH.   3.5 mIU/L (0.2–4.5)

TPO antibodies negative

Bridget is asymptomatic.

What would you like to ask the patient?

• The patient has unusual TFT results with elevated FT4, normal T3 without suppression of TSH

• Drug history should be established (is the patient on thyroxine or other treatment that may alter thyroid function?)

Bridget denies ever taking any thyroxine. Her medication includes: amiodarone (started 3 months ago), warfarin, ibuprofen and paracetamol

Can you explain her abnormal TFTs now?

• Amiodarone use can impair thyroid function in a number of ways

  ○ It can result in abnormal TFTs, which have no clinical significance

  ○ It may cause clinical hyperthyroidism

  ○ It may result in clinical hypothyroidism

• Due to suppression of T4 to T3 conversion, amiodarone use can be associated with:

  ○ High FT4 concentrations, without clinical hyperthyroidism (therefore, it is essential to check T3 in patients receiving amiodarone treatment)

  ○ Low FT3 concentrations (usually low normal levels)

○ In the first 3 months of amiodarone use, TSH may be elevated (lack of full negative feedback on the pituitary due to low T3 levels)

○ After 3 months, the pituitary seems to adjust to the low normal T3 concentrations and TSH normalizes

The combination of high FT4, normal T3 and TSH in an individual taking amiodarone is not uncommon and does not require any medical intervention at this stage, but will require regular monitoring.

Bridget's repeat TFTs in 3 months show:

FT4   25.1 pmol/L

FT3   4.1 pmol/L

TSH   3.8 mIU/L

What would you do now?

• Nothing

• Keep monitoring TFTs every 3–6 months

Bridget is referred 18 months later by her GP with clear symptoms and signs of hyperthyroidism and TFTs showing:

FT4   67 pmol/L

FT3   19.1 pmol/L

TSH   <0.05 mIU/L

What do these results indicate?

Bridget now has frank primary hyperthyroidism as shown by:

• High thyroid hormones (both T3 and T4)

• Suppressed TSH

  Bridget has amiodarone-induced hyperthyroidism.

What other tests would you request?

• Thyroid autoantibodies

• CRP

• Thyroid ultrasound (Doppler studies)

  In type 1 AIT:

  ○ Thyroid antibodies are positive in the majority

  ○ CRP levels are usually normal

Endocrinology and Diabetes: Clinical Cases Uncovered. By R. Ajjan. Published 2009 by Blackwell Publishing, ISBN: 978-1-4051-5726-1

Table 36 Differentiation between type 1 and type 2 amiodarone-induced thyrotoxicosis (AIT).

	Type 1 AIT	Type 2 AIT
Clinical		
Goitre	Usually present	Absent
Blood tests		
Thyroid autoantibodies	Positive (majority)	Negative
Plasma CRP	Normal	Elevated
Doppler studies and RAI uptake		
Vascularity	Increased	Decreased
Radioiodine uptake	Normal or reduced	Absent
Treatment		
Antithyroid drugs	Yes	No
Steroids	No	Yes

> **Box 29 Amiodarone-induced hyperthyroidism**
>
> - Type 1 amiodarone-induced thyrotoxicosis (AIT): similar to autoimmune hyperthyroidism (increased production of thyroid hormones)
> - Type 2 AIT: similar to thyroiditis (thyroid destruction and release of thyroid hormones)
>   It is important to differentiate between the two types as they are treated differently (see Table 36). Some patients may have a mixed type, in which case they should be treated for both type 1 and type 2 AIT.

  ○ Thyroid ultrasound (Doppler) shows increased vascularity
In type 2 AIT:
  ○ Thyroid antibodies are usually negative
  ○ CRP levels are elevated
  ○ Thyroid Doppler shows decreased vascularity

Bridget's tests showed
TPOAb negative
CRP 56 mg/L
Ultrasound Doppler decreased vascularity

How would you treat the patient?

The patient's investigations are consistent with type 2 AIT and the treatment includes:
- Discontinuation of amiodarone if possible
- High-dose oral steroids (prednisone 40 mg daily.)

The cardiologists are keen to continue amiodarone treatment and Bridget is started on steroids for 4 weeks followed by a reducing dose. Her TFTs 3 months later (off steroids) showed:
FT4   21.1 pmol/L
FT3   4.6 pmol/L
TSH   3.9 mIU/L.

What do these results indicate?

The patient is now euthyroid and no action is required other than regular monitoring of her TFTs.

Bridget is seen 3 months later with the following TFTs:
FT4   12.1 pmol/L
FT3   3.8 pmol/L
TSH   10.1 mIU/L
She is clinically asymptomatic.

What would you do?

- The blood tests are consistent with subclinical hypothyroidism
- The patient is likely to become clinically hypothyroid (which is not uncommon after type 2 AIT, due to thyroid destruction)
- As she is clinically asymptomatic, no treatment is necessary at this stage (just in case her thyroid recovers) and she can be simply followed up with repeat TFTs

She is seen 3 months later with TFTs:
FT4   6.7 pmol/L
FT3   1.6 pmol/L
TSH   39.2 mIU/L
Clinically, she has classical symptoms of hypothyroidism.

What would you do?

Bridget's TFTs are consistent with hypothyroidism and she should, therefore, start treatment on thyroxine.

Box 30 Amiodarone facts

- Amiodarone has a high iodine concentration (40% of weight), which contributes to the abnormal TFTs seen during treatment with this drug
- More than a quarter of patients taking amiodarone develop abnormalities in thyroid function
- Up to 5% of patients develop clinical hyperthyroidism and up to 15% develop clinical hypothyroidism

- Amiodarone-induced hyperthyroidism can develop a few months after stopping amiodarone due to the long half-life of the drug
- Differentiating type 1 from type 2 AIT can be difficult, in which case the patient should be treated for both with high-dose antithyroid drugs and steroids

---

CASE REVIEW

Bridget, who is on amiodarone treatment for paroxysmal atrial fibrillation, has abnormal thyroid function with elevated levels of T4, whereas T3 and TSH are normal. Amiodarone can affect the thyroid gland and cause hypothyroidism, hyperthyroidism and may also result in mildly abnormal TFTs, which have no clinical significance. Due to inhibition of T4 to T3 conversion in the periphery, amiodarone resulted in the initial abnormal thyroid function seen here, and this has no clinical significance. However, 18 months later Bridget developed symptoms of hyperthyroidism and her thyroid function was consistent with frank hyperthyroidism (raised T3, T4 and suppressed TSH). The differential diagnosis is between type 1 amiodarone-induced thyrotoxicosis (similar to autoimmune hyperthyroidism) or type 2 (similar to thyroiditis). Her investigations showed negative thyroid antibodies, raised CRP and reduced thyroid gland vascularity consistent with type 2 amiodarone-induced thyrotoxicosis. She was treated with steroids and her thyroid function normalized after 3 months. Subsequently, she became hypothyroid (low FT4 and raised TSH) secondary to thyroid tissue destruction following her thyroiditis and was started on treatment with thyroxine.

KEY POINTS

- Amiodarone, which has a high iodine content, can cause hypothyroidism (around 15% of patients), hyperthyroidism (around 5% of patients) and can result in abnormal thyroid function (high T4 with or without high TSH and normal T3), which has no clinical significance
- Amiodarone-induced thyrotoxicosis (AIT) can be divided into
  - AIT type 1: similar to autoimmune hyperthyroidism and usually characterized by presence of a goitre, positive thyroid antibodies, increased vascularity of the thyroid gland on Doppler examination and response to antithyroid drugs
  - AIT type 2: similar to thyroiditis and usually characterized by no goitre, raised CRP levels, decreased vascularity of the thyroid gland and response to steroid treatment
  - Mixed AIT: a mixture of type 1 and type 2 and is treated by both steroid and antithyroid agents
- It is preferable to stop amiodarone in AIT if at all possible
- Amiodarone-induced hypothyroidism is simply treated with thyroxine replacement
- Patients on amiodarone treatment should be regularly monitored for the development of thyroid dysfunction

Case 15 A 22-year-old man with hypertension

Stuart, who is 22 years old, is found to be hypertensive at 188/105 during routine blood pressure measurement taken after registering with a new GP. The patient is asymptomatic and there is no previous history of note. Two repeat blood pressure measurements in the next few days showed readings of 185/103 and 182/101.

What is the differential diagnosis at this stage?

The patient has high blood pressure. This can be divided into:

- Essential hypertension: majority of cases
- Secondary hypertension: this should be considered here due to the patient's young age. Causes of secondary hypertension include:
  - Renal disease: parenchymal or vascular (renal artery stenosis)
  - Coarctation of the aorta
  - Endocrine abnormalities: pheochromocytoma, primary aldosteronism, Cushing's syndrome, acromegaly, associated with primary hyperparathyroidism

What would be your next step?

- A thorough history
- Physical examination

What symptoms would you look for?

- Chronic renal disease
  - Fatigue
  - Muscle cramps
  - Itchy skin
- Coarctation of the aorta
  - Symptoms of heart failure
- Pheochromocytoma
  - Episodes of palpitations

Endocrinology and Diabetes: Clinical Cases Uncovered. By R. Ajjan. Published 2009 by Blackwell Publishing, ISBN: 978-1-4051-5726-1

  - Sweating and heat intolerance
  - Episodes of pallor
  - Headaches
- Primary aldosteronism (symptoms of hypokalaemia)
  - Weakness
  - Paraesthasia
  - Cramps
- Cushing's syndrome
  - Weight gain
  - Easy bruising
  - Abdominal striae
  - Visual problems (in case of pituitary adenoma)
- Acromegaly
  - Headaches
  - Increased sweating
  - Change in shoe and glove sizes
  - Visual problems

What signs would you look for during physical examination?

- Signs of renal disease
- Abdominal bruits (renal artery stenosis)
- Radio-femoral delay; weak or absent femoral pulses; cardiac murmurs (coarctation of the aorta)
- Abdominal masses (pheochromocytoma)
- Signs of Cushing's syndrome
- Signs of acromegaly
- Signs of hypertensive retinopathy

The patient has a normal physical examination except for grade II hypertensive changes on funduscopy. His ECG is shown in Fig. 57.

What is the significance of this ECG?

- It shows left ventricular hypertrophy, indicating long-standing and severe hypertension
- LVH on ECG and retinal changes indicate end organ damage secondary to hypertension

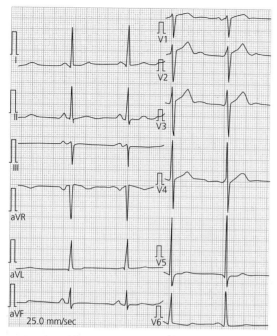

Figure 57

What investigations would Stuart need at this stage?

- U&Es, to rule out chronic renal disease
- Calcium profile
- CXR: may show signs of coarctation of the aorta
- Renal ultrasound and renal artery Doppler or magnetic resonance angiography (MRA) to rule out renal artery stenosis
- Urinary catecholamines (rule out pheochromocytoma)
- If there is any suspicion of Cushing's syndrome
  - 24 h urinary cortisol
  - Overnight or low-dose dexamethasone suppression test
- If there is any suspicion of acromegaly
  - Glucose tolerance test with GH measurement
- Thoracic MRI or CT should be arranged if there is suspicion of coarctation of the aorta

Stuart's tests showed:
Renal ultrasound and Doppler normal
Urinary catecholamines: normal on three occasions

Na	*144 mmol/L*
K	*3.0 mmol/L*
U	*5.4 mmol/L*
HCO$_3^-$	*29 mmol/L*
Creatinine	*76 μmol/L*
Calcium	*2.3 mmol/L*

What do these results indicate?

- These results rule out pheochromocytoma and chronic renal disease as the cause of this patient's hypertension
- Normal renal artery Doppler makes a diagnosis of renal artery stenosis highly unlikely although it does not conclusively rule out this diagnosis, which may require MRA in suspicious cases
- The combination of low potassium and high bicarbonate (hypokalaemic alkalosis) is strongly suggestive of primary aldosteronism as a cause of the hypertension in this patient
- Hypokalaemic alkalosis and hypertension may also occur in Cushing's syndrome and this should be ruled out if there is any clinical suspicion

What test would you request next?

- Potassium should be normalized with supplements followed by blood tests to check:
  - Plasma renin activity (PRA)
  - Aldosterone
- The patient should not be on any hypertensive medications that may interfere with PRA and aldosterone, such as:
  - ACEI
  - β-blockers
  - spironolactone
- If treatment of the patient is necessary while the above tests are carried out, α-blockers (i.e. doxazosin) or calcium channel-blockers can be used

Supine measurements of aldosterone and PRA are carried out and these show:

Aldosterone	*1220 nmol/L (100–500)*
PRA	*0.2 pmol/ml/hr (1.1–2.7)*

What do these results indicate?

The diagnosis is probable primary hyperaldosteronism resulting in hypertension and this is supported by:
- High aldosterone levels
- Low PRA

A ratio of aldosterone/PRA >2000 is diagnostic of primary aldosteronism.

What radiological test would you request and why?

- MRI of the adrenal glands
- Primary aldosteronism may be due to:
  - Adrenal adenoma (usually benign): this can be treated surgically or medically
  - Adrenal hyperplasia: no role for surgical intervention and treatment is medical

MRI shows a nodule in the left adrenal gland measuring 2.4 cm in diameter.

What is the most likely diagnosis?

The most likely diagnosis is Conn's syndrome (adrenal adenoma secreting excessive aldosterone).

What treatment would you advise?

- Surgical removal of the adrenal adenoma is advised
- It should be noted that large tumours (more than 4 cm in size) have a greater potential of being malignant and these should always be surgically removed

The patient asks you 'Would my high blood pressure be cured after having surgery?'

Hypertension is cured in only two-thirds of patients with Conn's syndrome following surgical removal of the tumour and this should be made clear to the patient.

What medical treatment can you offer?

- Spironolactone (aldosterone antagonist): side effects include gynaecomastia and impotence in men, menstrual irregularities in women
- Potassium-sparing diuretic
  - Amiloride
  - Triamterene

PART 2: CASES

CASE REVIEW

Stuart is a young man who is found to be hypertensive during routine examination. Subsequent measurements of blood pressure confirm a diagnosis of hypertension. Due to his young age, secondary hypertension is suspected. Apart from retinal hypertensive changes, his clinical examination is unremarkable. His ECG shows left ventricular hypertrophy indicating end organ damage despite his young age. Initial investigations rule out renal artery stenosis and pheochromocytoma, but hypokalaemic alkalosis suggests hyperaldosteronism as a cause of hypertension. This suspicion is confirmed by demonstrating a raised aldosterone:renin ratio and MRI imaging shows an adrenal tumour consistent with a diagnosis of Conn's syndrome. Surgical treatment is the best option for this condition although it does not normalize blood pressure in all patients. Medical treatment includes the aldosterone antagonist spironolactone and potassium-sparing diuretics (amiloride and triamterene).

KEY POINTS

- Secondary causes of hypertension should be suspected in young individuals and those with severe disease
- Secondary causes of hypertension include:
  - Kidney disease: vascular (renal artery stenosis) or parenchymal (chronic renal failure)
  - Endocrine disease: pheochromocytoma, primary aldosteronism, Cushing's syndrome, acromegaly
  - Cardiovascular disease: coarctation of the aorta
- Primary hyperaldosteronism should be suspected in individuals with hypertension and hypokalaemic alkalosis
- Diagnosis of primary hyperaldosteronism is usually confirmed by demonstrating raised aldosterone/renin activity (provided the patient is not on treatment with diuretics or agents that affect the renin-aldosterone system)
- Primary aldosteronism may be due to:
  - Adrenal adenoma (Conn's syndrome): usually treated with surgery
- Adrenal hyperplasia: treated medically
- Medical treatment of primary hyperaldosteronism includes:
  - Aldosterone antagonists: spironolactone
  - Potassium-sparing diuretics: amiloride and triamterene

Case 16   A 20-year-old woman with polyuria and polydipsia

Ivy, a 29-year-old woman, presents with a short history of polyuria and polydipsia.

What differential diagnosis would you be thinking of?

The differential diagnosis includes:

- Diabetes mellitus
- Hypercalcaemia
- Chronic renal failure
- Diabetes insipidus
- Psychogenic polydipsia

Her blood tests done by her GP earlier showed:

Glucose	20 mmol/L
Sodium	131 mmol/L
Potassium	4.4 mmol/L
Urea	5.4 mmol/L
Creatinine	76 μmol/L
Calcium	2.34 mmol/L

What questions would you ask this patient?

Ivy has high plasma glucose levels indicating a diagnosis of diabetes. It is important at this stage to differentiate between type 1 diabetes (T1DM) and T2DM. Questions to ask:

- How long have the symptoms of polyuria and polydipsia been present?
  - A short history of symptoms (days to weeks) is suggestive of T1DM
  - A long history of symptoms (months) or no symptoms is suggestive of T2DM
- History of rapid weight loss is strongly suggestive of T1DM

Endocrinology and Diabetes: Clinical Cases Uncovered. By R. Ajjan. Published 2009 by Blackwell Publishing, ISBN: 978-1-4051-5726-1

- Family history of diabetes
  - Family history of T1DM or autoimmunity (i.e. thyroid disease, pernicious anaemia) suggests a genetic predisposition to T1DM
  - Family history of diabetes at young age not requiring insulin or diabetes inherited in an autosomal dominant manner is suggestive of Maturity Onset Diabetes of the Young (MODY)

What test would you ask the nurse to perform that may help to differentiate between T1DM and T2DM?

Urine dipstick for ketones

- Heavy ketonuria is consistent with T1DM
- Absence of ketonuria does not rule out T1DM

What else would you like to know?

The weight/BMI of the patient

Box 31 Diabetes and BMI

- An overweight patient with diabetes is more likely to have T2DM
- A thin patient with diabetes is more likely to have T1DM
- However, T1DM can occur in obese individuals and T2DM may be seen in thin subjects

---

Ivy tells you that she had osmotic symptoms for 7–10 days, associated with 4 kg weight loss. Her sister has vitiligo but there is no other family history of note. Her BMI is 22 kg/m². Her urine dipstick shows:

Glucose 3+

Ketone 3+

Nitrate negative

WBC negative

What is the most likely diagnosis?

The most likely diagnosis is T1DM supported by:

- Short history of symptoms
- Significant weight loss
- Thin patient
- Family history of autoimmunity (vitiligo)

In unclear cases, can you do a blood test to help to differentiate between T1DM and T2DM?

- Glutamic acid decarboxylase (GAD) and islet cell antibodies are positive in the majority of T1DM patients (around 80%)
- A negative antibody test does not rule out the diagnosis of T1DM

What treatment would you start?

Ivy should be immediately started on insulin.

- Most patients can be managed on an out-patient basis.
- Admission should be considered for patients who look unwell or in the presence of abdominal pain/vomiting to rule out the possibility of diabetic ketoacidosis

---

Box 32 Insulin regimes

There are a number of insulin regimes, and the most commonly used are:

- Two injections a day with a mixture of insulin (short acting and long acting) such as:
  - Insulin aspart and aspart protamine (Novorapid 30)
  - Insulin lispro and lispro protamine (Humalog 25)
- Insulin actrapid and isophane (M3)
(the number indicates the percentage of short acting insulin in the mixture)
- Four injections a day, to include:
  - One injection of long acting insulin such as: insulin isophane (Insulatard), insulin glargine (Lantus) or insulin detemir (Levemir)
  - Three injections of short acting insulin that can be taken with meals: insulin aspart (Novorapid) or insulin lispro (Humalog)
- Although the second regime includes more injections, it gives more flexibility and is usually preferred for younger patients with diabetes

---

Ivy is started on Novomix 30, 12 units in the morning and 6 units in the evening and the dose is gradually titrated up to 24 and 14 units over a period of 6 weeks. Her glycaemic control was initially very good on these doses of insulin, but 4 months after diagnosis she had to drastically reduce the dose of her insulin to 8 and 4 units due to recurring hypoglycaemic attacks.

Why did this happen?

The pancreas of patients with T1DM may partially recover after the initial diagnosis resulting in decreased insulin requirement. This is known as the honeymoon period.

What do you need to ensure with any diabetes patient during a routine review?

- Ensure adequate control of blood sugar
  - Measure HbA1c levels and aim for <6.5%
  - Check glucose diary
- Look for signs of microvascular disease:
  - Eyes: retinopathy (retinal screening once a year)
  - Kidney: check for microalbuminuria (request urinary albumin/creatinine ratio once a year)
  - Feet: examine for neuropathy (monofilament test and vibration sense once a year)
- Ensure prevention/treatment of macrovascular complications:
  - Treat hypertension
  - Treat hyperlipidaemia: patients with diabetes above the age of 40 are usually started on lipid lowering treatment with a statin no matter what their plasma cholesterol levels are
  - Antiplatelet treatment (aspirin or clopidogrel) in high risk subjects
  - Aggressive measures for prevention/treatment from macrovascular disease should be implemented in the presence of microvascular complications

What are the types of diabetes?

The two main types of diabetes are shown in Table 20, p. 48. Traditionally, young patients with diabetes were more likely to have T1DM. However, due to the recent problem of obesity, T2DM can be now seen at a very young age (even children).

Other types of diabetes include:

- Maturity Onset Diabetes of the Young (MODY, up to 3% of T2DM)
  - This is a monogenic form of diabetes (due to a single gene defect)
  - Has an autosomal dominant mode of inheritance

o Patients are usually young and can be misdiagnosed as having T1DM
- Latent Autoimmune Diabetes of Adults (LADA)
  o An autoimmune form of diabetes occurring at an older age
  o Patients are usually slim
  o Patients are initially managed by oral hypoglycaemic agents but usually require insulin early after diagnosis (LADA is commonly a retrospective diagnosis)
- Gestational diabetes
  o Occurs during pregnancy
  o Disappears after giving birth
  o Subjects with a history of gestational diabetes are at increased risk of T2DM in the future
- Secondary diabetes
  o Destruction of the pancreas: pancreatitis, pancreatic tumour, infiltrative disease (haemochromatosis)
  o Endocrine abnormalities: acromegaly, Cushing's disease, pheochromocytoma, hyperthyroidism (rare)
- Associated with genetic syndromes
  o Down's syndrome
  o Turner's syndrome
  o Lawrence-Moon-Biedl syndrome
  o Prader-Willi syndrome
- Drug-induced
  o Steroids

Ivy's father, Andrew aged 62, presents a few months later to his GP, stating that his daughter checked his blood sugar with her glucose meter and found it to be elevated. He is asymptomatic and overweight with a BMI of 29.9. He has no past medical history of note and his urine dipstick shows:

Glucose 3+
Ketone   trace
Nitrate   negative
WBC   negative

What test would you request?

Fasting plasma glucose on two occasions.
- Diabetes is usually confirmed by checking fasting glucose twice, particularly in individuals who are asymptomatic
- In subjects with classical symptoms, one glucose sample is enough to confirm the diagnosis

His blood tests showed:
Fasting glucose: 10.3 and 11.6 mmol/L
HbA1c: 8.6%
U&Es   normal

What is the likely diagnosis?

This gentleman has T2DM supported by:
- High fasting plasma glucose (more than 7.0 mmol/L on two occasions)
- Overweight
- Absence of symptoms
- Urine dipstick negative for ketones

Rarely, some patients are misdiagnosed as having T2DM, when they have a secondary form of diabetes, and, therefore, the above list of causes of secondary diabetes should be kept in mind when assessing a new patient with suspected T2DM.

What medical treatment would you initiate to control his blood glucose levels?

None. Instead, advise the patient to:
- Change to a healthy diet
- Regular exercise
- Try to lose weight

Andrew implements your suggestions and is reviewed 3 months later. He has lost 4 kg in weight and his HbA1c is now 6.8%.

What would you do?

Congratulate Andrew and encourage him to continue with his programme of:
- Diet
- Exercise

He is reviewed 18 months later. Despite continuing with diet and exercise, his HbA1c has risen to 8.1%.

What would you do to control his blood sugar?

Andrew needs to be started on antidiabetic treatment. The preferred first-line agent in overweight T2DM patients is metformin (Glucophage).

Andrew is well on metformin for 2 years but his diabetes control subsequently deteriorates and his HbA1c rises to 8.9%.

What would you do now?

Andrew can be started on one of the following drugs:
- A sulphonylurea: this group of drugs stimulate insulin

> **Box 33 Common side effects of metformin**
>
> The most common side effects of metformin are gastrointestinal and include:
> - Nausea
> - Vomiting
> - Bloating
> - Diarrhoea
>
>   These side effects can usually be avoided by initiating a small dose of the drug and gradually titrating to higher doses. A long acting preparation of metformin (Glucophage SR) seems to be associated with fewer side effects.
>
>   The most serious side effect of metformin is lactic acidosis. This occurs in the presence of:
> - Renal failure
> - Advanced heart failure
> - Septicaemia
> - Therefore, metformin should be avoided in patients with a creatinine above 150 µmol/L or in those with *advanced* heart failure. Metformin should also be stopped in patients who become septic.

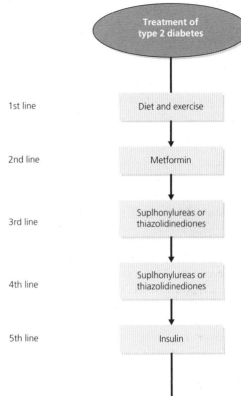

secretion by the pancreas. Commonly used drugs include:

- ○ Gliclazide
- ○ Glimepiride
- A thiazolidinedione: this group of drugs act as insulin sensitizers and seem to have cardioprotective properties. Commonly used drugs include:
  - ○ Rosiglitazone
  - ○ Pioglitazone

What are the two main drawbacks of sulphonylureas?

- Weight gain due to stimulation of insulin secretion
- Hypoglycaemia

What is the main contraindication for the use of thiazolidinediones?

- Heart failure is the main contraindication as these agents may cause fluid retention, thereby worsening existing heart failure

When do you use insulin in type 2 diabetes?

- Failure of oral therapy
- Hospital admission
  - ○ Infection
  - ○ Myocardial infarction

Figure 58 Treatment of type 2 diabetes. Metformin is usually the first-line agent except in those with contraindication or intolerance. Oral hypoglycaemic agents can be used in combination therapy (even as triple therapy). Insulin can be used in combination with metformin or a sulphonylurea and even pioglitazone. New agents that have been recently released include glucagon-like peptide analogues (injections) and DPP-4 inhibitors (oral), which can be used as second- to fourth-line agents.

- Pregnancy, as oral hypoglycaemics are contraindicated

Apart from antidiabetic agents, what other drugs are available that may help to control blood sugar?

- Slimming tablets such as:
  - ○ Sibutramine
  - ○ Orlistat
  - ○ Rimonabant
- Acarbose which inhibits glucose absorption
  Treatment of type 2 diabetes is summarized in Fig. 58.

CASE REVIEW

Ivy is a young woman presenting with a short history of polyuria and polydipsia. Her blood tests are consistent with a new diagnosis of diabetes. A detailed history is taken to establish the type of diabetes. A short history of symptoms in a lean patient, weight loss, a family history of autoimmunity and ketonuria all suggest a diagnosis of type 1 diabetes. In unclear cases, autoantibody measurement and insulin levels can be helpful to distinguish between different types of diabetes. Ivy is started on insulin treatment, which controls her diabetes well. However, her insulin requirements subsequently decrease due to partial recovery of the pancreas, often known as the honeymoon period, which is a temporary phenomenon.

Andrew, Ivy's father, measures his blood sugar using his daughter's glucose meter and his capillary glucose is found to be elevated. He is asymptomatic, overweight and his urine test shows absence of ketonuria. His fasting glucose is checked on two occasions (as he is asymptomatic) and

found to be elevated confirming a diagnosis of diabetes. Andrew is overweight, asymptomatic with no ketonuria consistent with a diagnosis of type 2 diabetes. Andrew initially manages to control his diabetes with diet, exercise and weight loss. His diabetes control deteriorates 18 months later and he is started on metformin treatment, which is the first-line agent in overweight T2DM patients. His diabetes control deteriorates again and, traditionally, either a sulphonylurea or a thiazolidinedione can be given at this stage. Newer agents, including GLP-1 analogues and DDP-4 inhibitors, can also be used as second-, third- or fourth-line treatments.

It should be remembered that the majority of diabetes patients develop vascular complications and it is important to treat a cluster of risk factors, rather than blood sugar alone, in these patients to prevent long-term complications. These risk factors include hypertension, microalbuminuria, dyslipidaemia and increased thrombosis potential.

KEY POINTS

- Diabetes mellitus, a common condition, is characterized by high blood glucose
- Diagnosis of diabetes
  - Elevated fasting glucose (>7 mmol/L) or postprandial glucose (>11.1 mmol/L) twice in the absence of symptoms or once in the presence of symptoms
  - Glucose tolerance test is warranted in unclear cases and in those with impaired fasting glucose (>6 mmol/L)
  - Most cases of diabetes (around 80–90%) are due to type 2 diabetes, usually secondary to increased insulin resistance, a condition closely associated with obesity
  - In a minority, diabetes is due to specific autoimmune destruction of β cells (type 1 diabetes)
  - Less common causes of diabetes include generalized pancreatic destruction (chronic inflammation, alcohol, trauma), endocrine conditions (acromegaly, Cushing's syndrome) and other rare conditions
- Type 1 diabetes is characterized by:
  - Occurrence in the younger population (peak age 12 years but can occur at any age) and usually in individuals who are not overweight
  - Short history of osmotic symptoms (days to weeks)
  - Rapid weight loss
  - Ketonuria

- Type 2 diabetes is characterized by:
  - Occurrence in the older population (peak age 60 years but can occur at any age) and usually in individuals who are overweight
  - Long history of symptoms (months and even years) or no symptoms at all
  - No history of weight loss and no ketonuria
- Autoantibody testing (positive in the majority of type 1 diabetes) and fasting insulin levels (low or undetectable in type 1 diabetes) can help to distinguish type 1 from type 2 diabetes
- Treatment
  - Type 1 diabetes is treated with insulin and the most common regimes include: twice daily injections of mixed insulin (short acting and intermediate acting), four daily injections of long acting insulin (once) and short acting insulin with meals, insulin pump (continuous insulin infusion)
  - Type 2 insulin is treated in stepwise manner: step 1, diet and exercise; step 2, start metformin treatment; step 3, add in a sulphonylurea or thiazolidinedione; step 4, triple oral hypoglycaemic agent therapy; step 5, add in or switch to insulin treatment. Others: new agents (GLP-1 analogues and DDP-4 inhibitors can be used in

steps 2–4); consider weight-reducing agents (any step)
- A large proportion of diabetes individuals develop:
  ○ Microvascular complications (nephropathy, neuropathy and retinopathy)
  ○ Macrovascular complications (cardiovascular disease): major cause of mortality in diabetes
- In addition to glucose control, prevention of diabetic complications involves the management of a cluster of risk factors:
  ○ Hypertension (antihypertensive agents)
  ○ Dyslipidaemia (statins)
  ○ Microalbuminuria (ACE inhibitors and angiotensin receptor blockers (ARBs))
  ○ Increased coagulation potential (antiplatelet agents)

Case 17 A 78-year-old man with pain in the leg and knee

Graham, aged 78, has been undergoing investigations for pain in his right hip and knee. Routine blood tests showed:

Hb	13.4 g/L
WBC	8.7 × 10⁹/L
Plats	387 × 10⁹/L
Na	139 mmol/L
K	4.4 mmol/L
Urea	4.5 mmol/L
Creat	77 μmol/L
Glu.	5.4 mmol/L
ALT	28 U/L
AP	1370 U/L
GGT	31 U/L
Bil	16 μmol/L

How do you interpret these results and what would you do next?

• The only abnormality here is a high alkaline phosphatase (AP) with otherwise normal LFTs
• This suggests that raised AP is from a bony and not a liver origin
• If in doubt:
  ○ AP isoenzymes can be requested that can differentiate between AP of liver and bony origin
  ○ A raised AP with normal gamma glutamyl transpeptidase (GGT) further suggests that it is from a bony origin

What are the causes of raised bony AP?

• Osteomalacia
• Fractures
• Bony metastasis
• Paget's disease
• Growing children and adolescents

Endocrinology and Diabetes: Clinical Cases Uncovered. By R. Ajjan.
Published 2009 by Blackwell Publishing, ISBN: 978-1-4051-5726-1

How would you rule out osteomalacia in this patient?

Osteomalacia is associated with:
• Low or low-normal calcium
• Low vitamin D
• High PTH
• High AP

Therefore, calcium profile, vitamin D and PTH should be requested in this patient.

Calcium profile, vitamin D and PTH are all in the normal range.

What imaging would you request in this patient?

• X-ray of the hip and knee
• Isotope bone scan

Figure 59 shows a pelvic X-ray and bone uptake scan.

What abnormalities can you identify and what is the diagnosis?

• The X-ray shows mixed lytic and sclerotic bone lesions in the pelvic bone (particularly on the right)
• The bone scan shows multiple areas of increased uptake
  The likely diagnosis here is Paget's disease.

What are the common symptoms of Paget's disease?

• Up to 90% of individuals are asymptomatic and the disease is picked up during routine investigations for another pathology
• Symptoms include:
  ○ Bone pain
  ○ Bone deformity: bowing of the tibia is a classical sign
  ○ Nerve compression (may cause deafness)

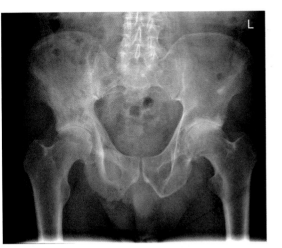

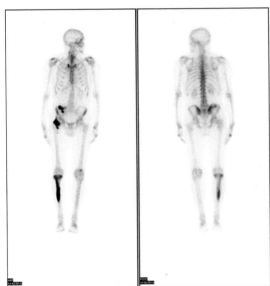

Figure 59 (a) X-ray of the hip lesions. (b) Bone uptake scan.

What are the signs of Paget's disease?

• Bone deformity (cranial and tibial bone deformity are classical features) (see Fig. 60, colour plate section, and Fig. 15)
• Warm bones due to the formation of collateral circulation
• A bruit can be heard over the bone secondary to extra blood flow
• Deafness (nerve compression)
• Cranial nerve palsies at the base of the skull
• Spinal cord compression
• Fractures
• Osteogenic sarcoma: rare and serious complication

Would you treat Graham and why?

Graham needs to be treated as he is:
• Symptomatic
• Has a high AP

What is the best treatment for this condition?

Bisphosphonates are currently the best treatment option for this condition.

How do you monitor response to treatment?

• Improvement in symptoms
• Reduction in AP levels

What happens to calcium levels in patients with Paget's disease?

Calcium levels are usually normal in uncomplicated Paget's disease.

What is the long-term management of this condition?

• Monitor for the development of complications
• Repeat bisphosphonate treatment as necessary

CASE REVIEW

Graham, who is 78 years old, presents with pain in his knee and leg. Initial investigations show a raised alkaline phosphatase with otherwise normal liver function tests. Calcium profile, vitamin D and parathyroid hormone levels are normal ruling out osteomalacia as a cause for raised alkaline phosphatase. Further investigations show bony destruction with new bone formation in the pelvis, whereas increased uptake in multiple bones is demonstrated on an uptake scan. These findings are consistent with a diagnosis of Paget's disease. The best treatment for symptomatic Paget's disease is bisphosphonate that can be given orally or intravenously.

KEY POINTS

- Paget's disease develops secondary to enhanced activity of osteoclasts, leading to increased osteoblast activity and disorganized new bone formation
- The commonest bones to be affected are:
  - Skull
  - Tibia
  - Pelvis
  - Vertebrae
- Clinically, Paget's disease is characterized by:
  - Bony pain
  - Bone deformity
  - The majority of patients are asymptomatic and the disease is picked up during routine investigations
- Diagnosis of Paget's disease is made by demonstrating:
  - Increased plasma levels of bony alkaline phosphatase
- X-ray findings consistent with bone resorption and new bone formation in a disorganized manner
- Bone uptake scan showing increased activity in affected areas
- Complications of the disease include:
  - Fractures
  - Deafness
  - Spinal cord compression
  - Development of osteogenic sarcoma: fortunately very rare
  - Hypercalcaemia
- Monitoring treatment
  - Clinical symptoms
  - Alkaline phosphatase levels

A 32-year-old woman with a lump in the neck

A GP refers Sharon with the following letter:
This 32-year-old woman has noticed a lump in her neck that moves with swallowing. An ultrasound examination confirmed this to be a thyroid nodule measuring 2 × 3 cm. I would be most grateful for your advice regarding the management of this patient's thyroid condition.

What specific questions would you like to ask the patient?

Questions asked should concentrate on trying to differentiate between a benign and malignant thyroid nodule. These should include the following:
- How long has the thyroid mass been there?
  - A long history (years) makes it unlikely to be malignant
- Has it been growing?
  - A mass that has not grown over the years is more likely to be benign
- Any associated symptoms?
  - Hoarseness and/or dysphagia may indicate a malignant condition spreading beyond the thyroid gland
- Previous history of radiation (particularly in childhood)
  - May raise the suspicion of a malignant condition
- Family history of thyroid cancer increases the risk of malignancy in a thyroid nodule
- Symptoms of hyperthyroidism
  - If the patient is thyrotoxic, the nodule *may be* hot (i.e. overactive), making it less likely to be malignant
- It is worth noting:
  - Thyroid nodules are more common in women but more likely to be malignant in men
  - Thyroid nodules are more likely to be malignant if the patient is younger than 20 or older than 60
  - The rate of malignancy in thyroid nodules is usually low (less than 10%)

- Malignant thyroid nodules are usually cold (non-functioning)

What would be your next step?
- Physical examination

What features would you be looking for during the physical examination?
- Establish the patient's thyroid status
- Neck examination to determine the characteristics of the nodule and feel for lymphadenopathy. Findings suggestive of malignancy include:
  - Firm or hard nodule
  - Fixation to adjacent tissue
  - Presence of lymphadenopathy

Sharon tells you that she noticed the nodule around 12 months ago and thinks that it may have grown in size in the past 2 months or so. On examination, the patient is clinically euthyroid and neck palpation reveals a firm solitary thyroid nodule with no fixation to adjacent tissue and she has no palpable lymph nodes. TFTs showed:
FT4   19.3 pmol/L
TSH   1.8 mU/L

What would be your next step?
Fine needle aspiration of the nodule.

Cytology of the fine needle aspiration of the thyroid is consistent with a papillary carcinoma.

What is the best treatment option for this patient?
- Surgery (total thyroidectomy)
- Radioiodine treatment is usually arranged after surgery for the ablation of any possible thyroid remnants

The patient undergoes thyroidectomy followed by radioiodine ablation. There is no evidence of tumour spreading beyond the thyroid gland.

Endocrinology and Diabetes: Clinical Cases Uncovered. By R. Ajjan.
Published 2009 by Blackwell Publishing, ISBN: 978-1-4051-5726-1

> ### Box 34 Different types of thyroid cancer
>
> - Papillary carcinoma
>   - Commonest (70–80%)
>   - Age at presentation: usually 30–50
>   - Prognosis: good
>   - Treatment: thyroidectomy and radioiodine remnant ablation
> - Follicular carcinoma
>   - Less common (15%)
>   - Age at presentation: usually 40–50
>   - Prognosis: good
>   - Treatment: thyroidectomy and radioiodine remnant ablation
> - Anaplastic carcinoma
>   - Rare (5%)
>   - Age at presentation: usually 60–80
>   - Prognosis: poor
>   - Treatment: surgery and chemotherapy
> - Lymphoma
>   - Uncommon
>   - Age at presentation: usually in women >40, with a background of Hashimoto's thyroiditis
>   - Prognosis: variable
>   - Treatment: radiotherapy/chemotherapy
> - Medullary thyroid carcinoma
>   - Rare: can be familial
>   - Age at presentation: any age (may even occur in children particularly as part of multiple endocrine neoplasia type 2)
>   - Prognosis: variable
>   - Treatment: surgery

What is the prognosis in this case?

Prognosis is excellent with more than 95% cure rate in developed countries.

After surgery and radioiodine ablation, Sharon is treated with thyroxine replacement with a dose of 150 mcg/day. Her TFTs showed:

FT4   20.3 pmol/L

TSH   1.2 mIU/L

What would you do?

- TSH stimulates the growth of benign as well as malignant thyroid cells
- Therefore, in patients post-thyroidectomy for papillary or follicular cancer, thyroxine replacement should aim to suppress TSH without inducing clinical thyrotoxicosis

- Therefore, the dose of thyroxine replacement should be increased to suppress TSH levels, without causing significant clinical thyrotoxicosis
- TSH suppression is not necessary in patients with medullary thyroid cancer or those with lymphoma, as the malignant cells are not TSH responsive (they are not thyroid follicular cells)

How would you monitor patients with treated thyroid cancer?

- Regular physical examination
- Thyroglobulin measurement in the plasma:
  - Detection of thyroglobulin in a patient who had previous thyroidectomy and ablation therapy indicates the presence of thyroid tissue
  - This is particularly important if thyroglobulin becomes measurable following a period when levels of this protein were undetectable

If our patient was both clinically and biochemically thyrotoxic on presentation, what would you have done?

- In a patient who is thyrotoxic and with a thyroid nodule, we need to establish whether:
  - The patient has a toxic (hot) nodule causing thyrotoxicosis (unlikely to be malignant)
  - The patient has an overactive thyroid (Graves' disease or toxic goitre) with a cold nodule (cold

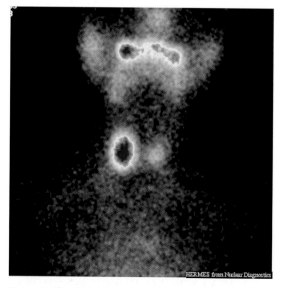

Figure 61 Thyroid uptake scan.

nodules are more likely to be malignant in patients with Graves' disease)

- The patient should, therefore, undergo a thyroid uptake scan to differentiate between the two above possibilities

I *Figure 61 is a thyroid uptake scan from a thyrotoxic patient.*

What does it show?

- A hot nodule (increased uptake), in the right lobe of the thyroid

What are the complications of thyroidectomy?

- Hypothyroidism
- Hypocalcaemia (secondary to damage of the parathyroid glands)
- Recurrent laryngeal nerve damage (resulting in a hoarse voice)
- Local haemorrhage
- Wound infection
- Keloid formation

CASE REVIEW

Sharon, a young woman, is referred by her GP for advice regarding the management of a thyroid nodule. This is a common condition and fortunately most thyroid nodules are benign. Clinical features suggestive of malignancy include a fast growing and hard nodule, hoarseness of voice or dysphagia and the presence of cervical lymphadenopathy. Special care should be taken in individuals with a previous history of irradiation or a family history of thyroid cancer. Thyroid nodules can be functional, secreting excess thyroid hormone, which are very rarely malignant, whereas non-functional nodules may be malignant. A thyroid uptake scan is helpful to distinguish between cold (non-functional) and hot (producing excess thyroid hormones) nodules in individuals who are thyrotoxic. Sharon was found to be euthyroid and, therefore, she has undergone a fine needle aspiration of the thyroid nodule, which was consistent with a papillary thyroid carcinoma. Consequently, she was referred for surgery followed by radioiodine ablation, which is a standard treatment regime for papillary thyroid carcinoma. The prognosis for this type of thyroid cancer, which is the commonest, is very good with a cure rate approaching 95%.

KEY POINTS

- Thyroid nodules are common, with a prevalence rate of 5–30% according to the population studied (prevalence in the UK is around 10%)
- Only a minority of thyroid nodules are cancerous and these are usually non-functional
- Toxic thyroid nodules are very unlikely to be malignant
- Special care should be taken in individuals with a previous history of irradiation or a family history of thyroid cancer (malignancy more likely)
- Clinical features of malignant thyroid nodules include:
  - Fast growing, hard nodules and skin fixation over the nodule
  - Presence of cervical lymphadenopathy
  - Hoarseness of voice
  - Dysphagia
- In euthryoid individuals, the first-line investigation of a thyroid nodule is fine needle aspiration
- In an individual with thyrotoxicosis and thyroid nodule(s), thyroid uptake scan should be arranged to investigate whether the nodule(s) are cold (non-functional) or hot

(producing excess thyroid hormones). A toxic nodule is usually benign, whereas cold nodule in an individual with Graves' disease carries a significant risk of malignancy
- Thyroid cancers include:
  - Papillary (75%)
  - Follicular (10%)
  - Medullary (5%)
  - Anaplastic (5%)
  - Lymphoma (5%)
- The prognosis of papillary and follicular thyroid cancers is usually good, whereas anaplastic cancers carry a very poor prognosis. Medullary cancers and lymphomas have a variable prognosis
- Treatment of thyroid cancers involves:
  - Surgery and radioiodine ablation therapy (papillary and follicular)
  - Surgery (medullary)
  - Radiotherapy and chemotherapy (lymphoma)
  - Palliative radiotherapy (anaplastic)
- It important to give a high dose of thyroxine replacement

Continued

to suppress TSH in patients with previous papillary and follicular thyroid cancers, without rendering them clinically thyrotoxic

- Patients with previous thyroid cancer should have lifelong monitoring in specialist centres, using:
  - Clinical examination
  - Thyroglobulin measurement (increased levels in disease relapse)
  - Imaging in cases of clinical suspicion: thyroid uptake scan, neck ultrasound, magnetic resonance imaging

Case 19 A 26-year-old with headaches and hypertension

Omar, who is 26 years old, is seen by his GP because of recurrent headaches and generally feeling unwell. His blood pressure was found to be elevated at 195/100.

What would you do next?

Secondary causes of hypertension should be sought (detailed in Case 15) and appropriate history and physical examination should be undertaken.

The patient tells you that for the past 6 months, he has been suffering from increased sweating and heat intolerance, severe headaches and episodes of palpitations associated with pallor.

From the history, what would you like to rule out as a cause for this patient's hypertension?

Given the:
- Symptoms
- Young age
- Severe hypertension
  A pheochromocytoma should be ruled out.

What test would you request?

Three 24-h urine collections for catecholamine and metanephrine measurement (see Part 1, p. 33).

Urinary catecholamines were found to be two- to threefold above the upper end of normal in all three 24-h urinary collections.

What would you do next?

The results are highly suggestive of a pheochromocytoma. The next step should be directed at localizing the tumour. Imaging techniques include:

Endocrinology and Diabetes: Clinical Cases Uncovered. By R. Ajjan. Published 2009 by Blackwell Publishing, ISBN: 978-1-4051-5726-1

- Abdominal MRI: sensitive at detecting these tumours
- CT: less sensitive at detecting adrenal tumours
- Radiolabelled meta-iodobenzylguanidine (MIBG) scan: this is positive in around three-quarters of pheochromcytomas and may detect tumours not visualized by MRI

The patient is found to have a large left adrenal tumour measuring 5 cm in diameter. The surgeon would like to immediately remove the tumour.

Do you agree?

- No, because a surgical procedure in a patient with a pheochromocytoma may precipitate a hypertensive crisis
- The patient should be prepared for surgery with appropriate antihypertensive therapy

What antihypertensive is used to treat these patients?

- Patients are usually treated with α-blockers (phenoxybenzamine)
- Before surgery, i.v. phenoxybenzamine is used for 3 days to ensure complete α-blockade
- β-blockers can only be used once the patient is fully α-blocked

The patient undergoes surgery and the tumour is successfully removed with restoration of normotension off any antihypertensive treatment. However, during routine tests, the patient's calcium is found to be elevated at 3.2 mmol/L.

What test would you request next?

Any patient with hypercalcaemia should have their PTH levels checked.

The patient's PTH levels are elevated at 14.3 pmol/L (normal range 1–6.1 pmol/L).

What is the cause of hypercalcaemia?

Raised calcium with raised PTH is indicative of primary hyperparathyroidism.

What diagnosis would you suspect in this case?

The combination of pheochromocytoma and primary hyperparathyroidism should raise the suspicion of multiple endocrine neoplasia type II (MEN II).

What other endocrine organ would you like to examine in this patient and why?

The thyroid gland should be examined in this patient as MEN II includes:

- Medullary thyroid cancer (MTC): often the initial presentation of this familial condition and it occurs in all individuals involved
- Pheochromocytoma: usually occurs later in up to half the affected individuals
- Hyperparathyroidism: occurs in around a quarter of the affected subjects

I *The patient is found to have a large thyroid nodule.*

What blood test(s) may help you to confirm your suspicion?

- The patient probably has a medullary thyroid carcinoma
- Serum calcitonin can be requested, which is usually elevated in patients with MTC

What is the aetiology of MEN II?

- MEN II is due to a mutation in the ret proto-oncogene, which is a transmembrane receptor
- Any patient who is suspected to have MEN II should be screened for a ret proto-oncogene mutation
- As MEN is an autosomal dominant condition, other family members should also be screened for the mutation

Are all pheochromocytomas familial?

No, only 10% are familial (some would argue up to 20% are familial). Familial pheochromocytomas can be seen in:

- MEN II
- Von Hippel-Lindau disease, which includes:
  - CNS and retinal haemangioblastomas
  - Pheochromocytoma
  - Renal cysts and carcinoma
- Neurofibromatosis type I, which includes:

- Multiple neurofibromas (Fig. 62, colour plate section)
- Café au lait spots
- Iris Lisch nodules
- Endocrine abnormalities including pheochromocytoma

Does a pheochromocytoma tumour always occur in the adrenal gland?

No, 10% can be extra-adrenal.

Can a pheochromocytoma occur in both adrenal glands?

Yes, 10% are seen in both adrenal glands.

Is pheochromocytoma a benign tumour?

Most are, but 10% can be malignant.

> **Box 35 Rule of 10 when dealing with a pheochromocytoma**
>
> The rule of 10 refers to the fact that approximately 10% of pheochromocytomas are:
> - Familial
> - Extra-adrenal
> - Bilateral
> - Malignant

What is MEN I?

MEN I is also an autosomal dominant condition secondary to a mutation in the menin gene. It involves the association of:

- Parathyroid hyperplasia
- Pancreatic endocrine tumours, usually:
  - Gastrinoma
  - Insulinoma
- Pituitary adenomas, usually:
  - Prolactinoma
  - Acromegaly
- MEN I is best remembered by PPP:
  - Parathyroid
  - Pancreas
  - Pituitary
- MEN II is best remembered by TAP:
  - Thyroid
  - Adrenal
  - Parathyroid

Patients and their relatives with MEN I or MEN II should be managed in specialized endocrine clinics with the help of a geneticist.

CASE REVIEW

Omar, a young man, visits his doctor with episodes of headaches, increased sweating, palpitations and is found to have significant hypertension. These symptoms raise the possibility of pheochromocytoma as the cause of his hypertension (secondary hypertension is discussed in Case 15). Further investigations demonstrate high levels of urinary catecholamines, indicating a diagnosis of pheochromocytoma. Imaging of the adrenal shows a 5-cm adrenal mass and the surgeon wants to undertake immediate surgery. However, Omar should be treated with α-blockers prior to surgery to lower the blood pressure and avoid a hypertensive crisis, which may occur during the operation. After appropriate medical management, Omar undergoes successful adrenal surgery but his calcium and PTH levels are found to be elevated after the operation, indicating a diagnosis of primary hyperparathyroidism. The association of pheochromocytoma and primary hyperparathyroidism should raise the suspicion of multiple endocrine neoplasia type II. This diagnosis is further supported by the presence of a thyroid nodule, likely to be a medullary carcinoma, in which case plasma calcitonin levels are elevated.

KEY POINTS

- Individuals with severe hypertension, particularly the young, should be investigated for the possibility of secondary hypertension (see Case 15)
- Pheochromocytomas are rare medullary adrenal tumours and a cause of hypertension in less than 0.1% of cases
- Pheochromocytomas may be an isolated condition or part of/associated with:
  ○ MEN type II
  ○ Neurofibromatosis type I
  ○ Von Hippel-Lindau syndrome
- Clinical presentation of pheochromocytoma includes:
  ○ Hypertension sometimes with postural hypotension
  ○ Episodes of palpitations and sweating
  ○ Flushing or pallor
  ○ Headaches and visual disturbances
- The rule of 10 in pheochromocytoma:
  ○ Bilateral in 10%
  ○ Extra-adrenal in 10%
  ○ Malignant in 10%
- Diagnosis of pheochromocytoma is made by demonstrating raised urinary catecholamines and/or metanephrines in the urine
- Surgical treatment is curative in the majority of patients. Blood pressure should be controlled before surgery and α-blockers are given prior to the introduction of other antihypertensive agents. Intravenous phenoxybenzamine is given for 3 days before surgery to ensure full α-blockade

PART 2: CASES

Case 20 Sweating, nausea and hand tremor in a 24-year-old woman

Eleanor, a thin 24 year old woman, is seen at clinic with a few weeks' history of episodes of sweating, sometimes associated with hand tremor and feeling nauseous. The symptoms are particularly pronounced in the morning, frequently occur after exercise and are always relieved by eating.

What differential diagnosis would you think of at this stage?

Sweating can be due to a number of conditions including:
- Thyrotoxicosis
- Pheochromocytoma
- Carcinoid syndrome
- Menopause
- Hypoglycaemia
- Psychological

What would you do next?

A detailed history is essential concentrating on symptoms of:
- Thyrotoxicosis (see Case 2)
- Pheochromocytoma (see Case 19)
- Carcinoid syndrome (see Case 24)
- Early menopause: if periods are regular, this diagnosis is unlikely
- Hypoglycaemia: the fact the symptoms are relieved by eating suggests that this may be a possibility
- Psychological: this is only considered once the above possibilities are ruled out

Eleanor further tells you that her brother has type 1 diabetes and in view of this her GP checked her fasting blood glucose, which was found to be low at 2.2 mmol/L.

Endocrinology and Diabetes: Clinical Cases Uncovered. By R. Ajjan.
Published 2009 by Blackwell Publishing, ISBN: 978-1-4051-5726-1

What would you do next?

This suggests that the cause of this patient's symptoms is hypoglycaemia, which may be due to:
- Insulinoma
  - Usually a pancreatic tumour secreting insulin (benign in 85% of cases)
  - Diagnosis is made by demonstrating raised insulin levels and C peptide in the presence of hypoglycaemia
- Drug-induced
  - Insulin: injection of insulin in a non-diabetic individual results in hypoglycaemia, in which case plasma levels of insulin will be high but C peptide will be undetectable, in contrast to a patient with insulinoma. Insulin injection can be seen in: self-injection, patients with psychiatric problems (attention seeking and trying to commit suicide); and injection by others (possible criminal intent)
  - Sulphonylurea (both insulin and C peptide are elevated)
  - Alcohol (due to impairment of gluconeogenesis)
- Hormonal deficiencies:
  - Hypopituitarism
  - Addison's disease: tiredness, history of pigmentation (due to excessive ACTH secretion), weight loss and gastrointestinal symptoms (nausea and vomiting, abdominal pain, diarrhoea, dizziness and postural hypotension)
- In severely ill patients:
  - Organ failure (acute liver failure)
  - Infection (septicaemia, malaria)
- Postprandial
  - Usually postgastrectomy (dumping syndrome): rapid glucose absorption due to fast gastric emptying leads to excessive insulin secretion resulting in hypoglycaemia 1–3 h after eating
- Rare causes

◦ Autoimmune: insulin receptor activating antibodies

◦ Mesenchymal tumours secreting insulin-like growth factors

What are the symptoms of hypoglycaemia and what are they due to?

These can be divided into:

- Adrenergic
  ◦ Sweating
  ◦ Tremor
  ◦ Palpitation
  ◦ Pallor
- Neuroglycopenic (more likely to occur with prolonged hypoglycaemia)
  ◦ Poor concentration
  ◦ Confusion
  ◦ Irritability and uncharacteristic violent behaviours
  ◦ Seizures and coma in severe and more prolonged cases

On further questioning, Eleanor categorically denies insulin injection or sulphonylurea (SU) ingestion and her alcohol intake is less than 5 units a week. She has been feeling very tired for a few weeks, and has lost a stone in weight due to reduced appetite and nausea. She has also been feeling dizzy, particularly when getting out of bed first thing in the morning.

How would this information help you in the diagnosis?

Insulinoma is less likely as this condition is associated with weight gain; high insulin levels and hypoglycaemia result in frequent snacking.

- Drugs
  ◦ There is nothing in the history to suggest insulin/SU/alcohol as a cause of her hyperglycaemia
  ◦ However, most patients injecting insulin/taking SU deny ever doing so, often making the diagnosis a challenging task
- The patient is not severely ill (which would suggest organ failure or septicaemia as the cause for her symptoms)
- Hypoadrenalism (primary or secondary) is a possibility:
  ◦ Dizziness first thing in the morning is suggestive of postural hypotension, which is not infrequently seen in hypoadrenalism (more common in primary hypoadrenalism due to defective secretion of aldosterone)

◦ There is a family history of autoimmunity, and, therefore, Addison's disease is a possibility

Blood tests performed by the GP 10 days earlier showed:

Sodium	*131 mmol/L*
Potassium	*5.2 mmol/L*
Bicarbonate	*19 mmol/L*
Urea	*4.6 mmol/L*
Creatinine	*76 μmol/L*
Calcium	*2.62 mmol/L*

What is a possible diagnosis in this patient? What signs would you look for?

The patient has the following symptoms:

- Tiredness
- Weight loss
- Reduced appetite and nausea
- Probably postural hypotension
- Blood tests show:
  ◦ Fasting hypoglycaemia
  ◦ Hyponatraemia
  ◦ Hyperkalaemia
  ◦ Low bicarbonate
  ◦ Mild hypercalcaemia

A possible diagnosis is Addison's disease, which can be associated with the symptoms and the electrolyte abnormalities listed above.

Signs to look for include:

- Postural hypotension
- Pigmentation: seen only in primary hypoadrenalism (due to raised ACTH):
  ◦ Areas exposed to pressure (elbows, knees and under bras)
  ◦ Palmar creases
  ◦ Scar tissue
  ◦ Mucosa

On checking the blood pressure, a postural drop from 110/70 to 90/55 is noted. Eleanor has clear pigmentation in the oral mucosa and palmar creases.

What tests would you request next?

- Short synacthen test: serum cortisol is checked at 0 min and 30 min
- ACTH levels
- Plasma renin activity
- Aldosterone

Her blood tests showed:

Synacthen test:

0 min cortisol	*76 nmol/L*
30 min cortisol	*110 nmol/L*

ACTH 330 ng/L (normal range 10–80 ng/L)

Aldosterone   40 pmol/L (supine 100–500 pmol/L)

PRA   11.1 pmol/mL/h (supine 1.1–2.7 pmol/mL/h)

What is the diagnosis?

- The patient has a highly subnormal cortisol response to short synacthen test
- High ACTH
- Low aldosterone
- Elevated PRA

The diagnosis is, therefore, primary hypoadrenalism.

Box 36 Causes of primary hypoadrenalism

- Autoimmune: the commonest cause in Western society (more than two-third of cases)
- Vascular event: infarction or haemorrhage into the adrenal glands:
  - Antiphospholipid syndrome
  - Warfarin treatment
  - Meningococcal septicaemia (Waterhouse-Friedrichson syndrome)
- Infection
  - Tuberculosis
  - Fungal: histoplasmosis, cryptococcosis
  - Opportunistic infections: particularly in patients with AIDS
- Malignant metastatic disease
- Congenital adrenal hyperplasia
- Inherited disorders of fatty acid metabolism (adrenoleucodystrophy)
- Iatrogenic
  - Prolonged use of steroids followed by sudden withdrawal (adrenal glands may take some time to recover after suppression of function due to external steroids)
  - Ketoconazole: can suppress cortisol production (this drug is used to treat Cushing's syndrome)
  - Surgical adrenalectomy

What tests can be requested to establish the aetiology of this patient's hypoadrenalism?

- Serological
  - Adrenal autoantibodies, which are positive in most patients with autoimmune hypoadrenalism
- Radiological
  - CT or MRI of the adrenals
  - Adrenal enlargement can be seen in tuberculosis, infiltrative or metastatic disease
  - Adrenal atrophy is seen in autoimmune hypoadrenalism

Adrenal antibodies are positive and a diagnosis of autoimmune hypoadrenalism is made.

What treatment would you start and what precautions would you give the patient?

- Glucocorticoid replacement
  - Cortisol replacement divided into two or three daily doses
- Mineralocorticoid replacement
  - Fludrocortisone
- The patient should be advised to double the dose of steroids for a few days in case of a mild illness (i.e. cold or flu)
- If the patient is more severely ill, i.m. or i.v. steroids may be required
- The patient should be given an ampoule of hydrocortisone to inject in cases of emergency (i.e. unable to take oral steroids due to vomiting)

The patient is admitted 3 months later with:

Abdominal pain

Diarrhoea

Severe dizziness and low blood pressure at 60/40 mmHg.

What would you do?

The likely diagnosis is acute adrenal insufficiency. The patient should *immediately* be given:

- Intravenous steroids
- Intravenous fluids

In clinical practice, any patient with *unexplained hypotension* should be given a dose of hydrocortisone after taking a blood sample for random cortisol measurement.

CASE REVIEW

Eleanor is a young woman with a few weeks' history of episodes of sweating, hand tremor and feeling nauseous. These symptoms seem to occur in the morning or after exercise and are always relieved by eating, raising the possibility of hypoglycaemia as the cause. Hypoglycaemia may be due to insulinoma, which is usually associated with weight gain due to frequent snacking, excess alcohol, drugs (sulphonylurea abuse, insulin injections) and hypoadrenalism. The latter diagnosis is suspected due to symptoms of tiredness and weight loss as well as typical electrolyte abnormalities (hyponatraemia, hyperkalaemia with mildly low bicarbonate). In addition to confirming morning hypoglycaemia, Eleanor is found to have increased pigmentation in oral mucosa and palmar creases as well as postural hypotension, making the diagnosis of primary adrenal failure a strong possibility. This suspicion is confirmed by demonstrating an abnormal synacthen test, low aldosterone, together with elevated ACTH and plasma renin activity. Positive adrenal antibodies indicate autoimmune hypoadrenalism as the cause of adrenal failure, and this fits with a family history of autoimmunity. The patient should be treated with a combination of glucocorticoid and mineralocorticoid replacement and special precautions to double the dose of steroids in case of a mild illness and to give intravenous or intramuscular steroids in case of severe illness or if unable to take steroids orally (i.e. vomiting). Eleanor is admitted 3 months later with postural hypotension and gastrointestinal symptoms, suggesting acute adrenal insufficiency, also known as an adrenal crisis, which should be treated urgently with intravenous fluid and glucocorticoid.

KEY POINTS

- Hypoglycaemia should be suspected in individuals with episodes of nausea, hunger, sweating and tremor, particularly if symptoms are relieved by eating
- Causes of hypoglycaemia include:
  - Alcohol-induced
  - Insulinoma
  - Hypoadrenalism (primary or secondary)
  - Drug-induced: insulin or sulphonylurea
  - Reactive hypoglycaemia (occurs post meal, usually after gastric surgery)
  - Severe illness (septicaemia, liver failure)
  - Autoimmune (insulin or insulin receptor antibodies)
- Investigations of hypoglycaemia include:
  - Liver function tests
  - Ethanol concentration if alcohol abuse is suspected
  - Prolonged fasts (up to 72 h) with measurement of glucose, insulin and C peptide
  - Rule out adrenal insufficiency
- Treatment of hypoglycaemia:
  - Acute: conscious, oral glucose; unconscious, intravenous glucose and intramuscular glucagon
  - Chronic: treat the cause
- Hypoadrenalism should be suspected in individuals with:
  - Episodes of hypoglycaemia
  - Weight loss
  - Postural hypotension
  - Pigmentation of skin and buccal mucosa (primary hypoadrenalism)
- Causes of primary hypoadrenalism include
  - Autoimmune (majority of cases in the Western world)
  - Long-term steroid treatment
  - Infection (tuberculosis, fungal): particularly in the immunocompromised)
  - Vascular event (adrenal infarction or haemorrhage)
  - Infiltrative disease
  - Metastatic malignancy
  - Congenital adrenal hyperplasia
- Biochemical abnormalities in hypoadrenalism include:
  - Hyponatraemia
  - Hyperkalaemia
  - Mild metabolic acidosis
  - Anaemia and eosinophilia
  - Mild hypercalcaemia
- Diagnosis of primary adrenal failure is confirmed by demonstrating:
  - Subnormal cortisol response to short synacthen test
  - Raised ACTH levels
  - Low aldosterone with elevated plasma renin activity
  - Individuals with primary adrenal failure should be investigated for the cause

Case 21 A 19-year-old man with sexual dysfunction

Alex consults his GP, at the age of 19, with a history of sexual dysfunction.

What do you want to know at this stage?

Sexual dysfunction is a very common complaint, particularly in older men. Our patient is a young man and at this stage we need to establish:

• Is this an intermittent problem? The commonest cause of sexual dysfunction is non-organic (psychological) and an intermittent nature may be suggestive of this diagnosis
• Are there any associated stressful life events?
• In a young patient, history of pubertal development is essential:
  ○ Testicular size
  ○ Pubic hair
  ○ Body hair
  ○ Voice change
  ○ Penile development
• Previous history
  ○ Systemic illness (mumps can cause primary gonadal failure)
  ○ Testicular trauma
  ○ History of neurological disease: spinal cord disease, multiple sclerosis
  ○ History of vascular problems (usually in older patients)
  ○ Chemotherapy
  ○ Radiotherapy

On examination:
Height is 1.95 m (mother 1.67 m, father 1.76 m)
He has normal pubic and axillary hair distribution
He has little facial hair (shaves once every 5 days)

His testicles are small measuring 4–5 mL
He has a small penis measuring 3 cm in length and less than 2 cm in width
He has bilateral gynaecomastia

What do these findings suggest and what blood tests would you request at this stage?

• The patient is taller than expected (looking at the height of his parents)
• He has signs of delayed puberty
  ○ Small testicles
  ○ Underdeveloped penis
  ○ Little facial hair
• Blood tests to be requested next include
  ○ Testosterone
  ○ FSH and LH

His blood tests show:
Testosterone   5 nmol/L (normal range 10–40 nmol/L)
FSH   45 U/L (normal range 0.5–5 U/L)
LH   38 U/L (normal range 3–8 U/L)

What do these results suggest?

Primary gonadal failure supported by:

• Low testosterone
• Raised gonadotrophin

What other questions would you like to ask Alex at this stage?

• History of testicular trauma
• History of testicular infection or systemic illness as detailed above

There is no significant previous medical history.

What test would you like to request and why?

• Chromosomal analysis

Endocrinology and Diabetes: Clinical Cases Uncovered. By R. Ajjan. Published 2009 by Blackwell Publishing, ISBN: 978-1-4051-5726-1

Table 37 Differences in testicular failure occurring before and after puberty.

	Before puberty	After puberty
Testicular volume	<5 mL	<15 mL, soft
Penile length	<5 cm	Normal
Bone age	Delayed	Normal
Body hair	Greatly reduced	Some reduction
Voice	High pitched	Normal

○ A possible diagnosis here is Klinefelter's syndrome, which is the commonest cause of congenital primary hypogonadism, affecting around 1:500 men

What are the differences between testicular failure occurring before and after puberty?

These are summarized in Table 37. It should be noted that in some cases the distinction between these two entities is not that clear.

Alex's chromosomal analysis shows that the patient has an extra sex chromosome in XXY pattern.

What is the diagnosis?

The diagnosis is Kleinfelter's syndrome. The main clinical features of this syndrome include:

• Clinical
  ○ Sexual dysfunction
  ○ Reduced testicular volume
  ○ Gynaecomastia
  ○ Female type body composition (eunucoidism)
  ○ Intellectual dysfunction in around half the patients
• Biochemical
  ○ Low testosterone with high gonadotrophins
  ○ XXY karyotype
• Treatment
  ○ Androgen replacement: testosterone injections, testosterone gel, buccal testosterone, testosterone implants (rarely used now)

How do you advise this patient regarding fertility?

• Most Klinefelter's patients are infertile
• A minority can produce enough sperm to conceive, but this is rare

The patient's brother, Phil aged 41, with a 3-year history of T2DM presents with 10 months' history of erectile dysfunction. His blood tests show:

HbA1c	*6.8%*
ALT	*140 (normal range <40 IU/L)*
AP	*630 (normal range 100–300 IU/L)*
Bilirubin	*14 μmol/L*
Sodium	*143 mmol/L*
Potassium	*4.3 mmol/L*
Creatinine	*78 μmol/L*
Urea	*4.3 mmol/L*

What would you do now?

• Phil has good diabetes control supported by HbA1c <7%
• He has abnormal liver function manifested as raised ALT and AP
• A detailed history is essential, including:
  ○ Onset and severity: How long has he had the problem for? Is it intermittent? Can he achieve partial erection? An abrupt onset of erectile dysfunction, particularly one that is intermittent is often psychogenic in origin
  ○ Presence of night or morning erection: the absence of morning erection indicates an organic cause rather than a psychological problem
  ○ History of recent stress: which can be associated with erectile problems and decreased libido
  ○ Associated symptoms of androgen deficiency: reduced libido, reduced muscle strength, generally unwell and tired

Phil tells you that he has had the problem for around a year but can still achieve partial erection. Also, he noticed a decrease in libido in the past few months, which he thought might be related to his age. His medications include:
Metformin 850 mg twice daily
Simvastatin 40 mg daily
Aspirin 75 mg daily
He undergoes a full examination, which is recorded as normal.

What would you do now?

• A history of partial erection is very common in diabetes-related erectile dysfunction
• A decrease in libido may indicate reduced testosterone levels but may also occur during stressful life events
• None of his drugs are associated with erectile dysfunction. The drugs commonly associated with erectile dysfunction include:

○ Antihypertensives
○ Antidepressants
○ Tranquillizers
○ Steroid hormones
○ Alcohol
○ Heroin and marijuana
○ Digoxin
○ Anti-androgens

• Statin treatment may be responsible for the abnormal liver function and consideration should be given to stopping this treatment or reducing the dose

• Metformin treatment can also result in abnormal LFTs but this is less common

What tests in relation to erectile dysfunction would you request?

The following tests should be requested:

• Prolactin
• Testosterone
• FSH and LH

Blood tests show the following:

Prolactin	*211 mU/L (normal <600 mU/L)*
Testosterone	*5.6 nmol/L (normal range 10–40 nmol/L)*
FSH	*2.1 U/L (normal range 0.5–5 U/L)*
LH	*0.8 U/L (normal range 3–8 U/L)*

What do these tests show?

• Phil has hypogonadotrophic hypogonadism, supported by:
  ○ Testosterone levels are very low
  ○ FSH and LH levels are low

Are these results consistent with Klinefelter's syndrome?

No, in Klinefelter's gonadotrophins are high.

What other tests would you request here?

Full assessment of pituitary function to rule out deficiency of other pituitary hormones (see pp. 3 & 4).

Phil undergoes an insulin stress test. The results are shown in Table 38.
TFTs show:
FT4   16.7 pmol/L
TSH   2.4 mIU/L

Table 38 Results of insulin stress test.

	Glucose (mmol/L)	Cortisol (nmol/L)	Growth hormone (U/L)
0 min	5.1	360	1.2
30 min	5.3	410	1.5
60 min	2.8	530	5.9
90 min	1.6	740	12.1
120 min	1.8	810	25.6
150 min	4.1	820	26.2
180 min	5.2	790	26.3

How do you interpret these results?

• Insulin stress test shows adequate hypoglycaemia and appropriate elevation of cortisol and growth hormone (more than 580 nmol/L and 20 U/L respectively) ruling out ACTH and GH deficiency

• TFTs are normal, ruling out TSH deficiency

• Taken together, Phil has isolated FSH/LH deficiency as the cause of his hypogonadism

Would you request any imaging in this patient?

In view of secondary hypogonadism, pituitary MRI should be requested to rule out a primary pituitary pathology causing hypogonadotrophic hypogonadism.

MRI of the pituitary is normal. The GP requests one blood test that uncovers the aetiology of Phil's hypogonadism.

What is the aetiology?

Phil has:

• Diabetes
• Abnormal LFTs
• Hypogonadotrophic hypogonadism

Therefore, haemochromatosis should be ruled out and ferritin levels should be checked.

Phil's ferritin was very high at 1260 ng/mL (normal range 20–200 ng/mL).

What is the differential diagnosis of raised ferritin and what would you do for this patient?

The differential diagnosis for raised ferritin includes:

- Haemochromatosis
- Liver disease (including alcoholism)
- Cancers
- Autoimmune conditions

The patient should be referred to the haematologist for:

- Full assessment
- Treatment (usually venesection for haemochromatosis)
- Follow-up

The haematologists confirm a diagnosis of haemochromatosis.

How would you treat Phil's endocrine problem?

- If fertility is not an issue, simple testosterone replacement should be started
- If the patient wants to start a family, the treatment is more complicated with:
  - Human chorionic gonadotrophin (hCG; mimics LH action)
  - FSH

However, this therapy will not be successful if haemochromatosis has also affected the testicles (iron infiltration), in which case the patient will have a mixture of primary and secondary hypogonadism

What are the causes of secondary hypogonadism (i.e. associated with low gonadotrophin levels)?

- Infiltrative disease
  - Haemochromatosis
  - Histiocytosis
- Kallman's syndrome
  - A genetic disorder
  - Associated with anosmia in the majority of patients
- Idiopathic hypogonadotrophic hypogonadism (IHH)
- Functional
  - Excessive exercise
  - Stress
  - Recreational drugs
  - Systemic illness
  - Severe weight changes

> **Box 37 Causes of sexual dysfunction**
>
> **Endocrine causes**
> - Hypogonadism
>   - Primary
>   - Secondary
> - Thyroid dysfunction
> - Diabetes
> - Hyperprolactinaemia
>
> **Non-endocrine causes**
> - Drugs
> - Neurological disorders
>   - Spinal cord disease
>   - Multiple sclerosis
> - Vascular disease (generalized atherosclerosis)
> - Penile abnormalities
> - Psychogenic

CASE REVIEW

Alex, aged 19, is complaining of sexual dysfunction. Although this is a common problem with advancing age, it is relatively rare in this age group. A careful history and appropriate physical examination is important to help reach a correct diagnosis. On examination, Alex is found to be tall with little facial hair and small testicles and penis, together with bilateral gynaecomastia. His blood tests are consistent with primary testicular failure. Taken together, a likely diagnosis is Klinefelter's syndrome, which is confirmed on chromosomal analysis showing XXY karyotype. Testosterone replacement should be started in this patient and issues with fertility discussed as almost all individuals with Klinefelter's are infertile.

The patient's brother, Phil, a middle-aged gentleman with T2DM, also presents with a history of erectile dysfunction. This is a common problem in individuals with diabetes secondary to neuropathic changes and vascular disease. A detailed history does not give specific clues and his medications do not seem to be the cause. His blood tests are consistent with secondary gonadal failure

Continued

(low testosterone and inappropriately low/low normal gonadotrophins). His liver function is abnormal, which may be due to his treatment (statin) but can also be secondary to other pathologies. He undergoes investigations of the pituitary axis, and this shows normal cortisol and growth hormone response, whereas his prolactin levels and thyroid functions are normal, indicating isolated gonadotrophin deficiency. Further investigations show normal pituitary MRI but elevated ferritin levels. This suggests haemochromatosis as a unifying diagnosis for this patient's hypogonadotrophic hypogonadism (pituitary deposition of iron), abnormal liver function (liver deposition) and diabetes (pancreatic deposition). In addition to venesection, Phil will require testosterone or gonadotrophin replacement (the latter is only used when fertility is an issue).

KEY POINTS

- Erectile dysfunction is common, particularly in older individuals, and may be caused by neurological damage, vascular pathology, androgen deficiency and certain medications. It can also be psychological.
- Sexual history is important to establish the correct diagnosis, including:
  - Onset and progression (sudden onset erectile dysfunction is usually psychological)
  - Extent of the problem (partial or complete)
  - Presence of morning erections
  - Associated medical conditions (vascular disease, diabetes, spinal cord injuries)
  - Medications
  - Social history including recent stress, alcohol, recreational drugs
- Examination should include:
  - Hair distribution
  - External genitalia
  - Evidence of associated endocrine or other medical conditions
- Initial investigations for erectile dysfunction should include:
  - Testosterone, FSH and LH
  - Prolactin
  - Thyroid function tests
  - Fasting glucose
  - Renal and liver function tests
- Klinefelter's syndrome (KS) is the commonest congenital cause of primary hypogonadism and is characterized by:
  - Tall stature
  - Intellectual dysfunction in up to half the patients
  - Reduced testicular volume
  - Gynaecomastia
- Abnormal blood tests in KS include:
  - Low testosterone and raised gonadotrophins (primary gonadal failure)
  - Karyotype: usually XXY
- Other causes of primary hypogonadism include:
  - Testicular trauma or inflammation (mumps)
  - Chemotherapy or radiotherapy
  - Alcohol excess
  - Certain drugs
  - Cryptorchidism
  - Chronic illnesses (renal failure, liver cirrhosis)
- Causes of secondary hypogonadism:
  - Kallman's syndrome (frequently associated with anosmia)
  - Idiopathic hypogonadotrophic hypogonadism
  - Functional (stress, exercise, weight loss, acute systemic illness)
  - Any pituitary pathology
- Treatment of hypogonadism
  - Primary: testosterone replacement
  - Secondary: testosterone replacement (fertility is not a concern); gonadotrophin replacement (to restore fertility)

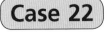

Case 22   A 38-year-old woman with muscular aches and weakness

Ayesha is a 38-year-old Asian woman who presents with a 2-month history of generalized muscular aches and weakness, in addition to feelings of pins and needles in her hands. Also, she is complaining of difficulties in standing up from a squatting position.

What would you do?
- Generalized aches and pain is a non-specific symptom and can be due to:
  - Muscle strain after exertion
  - Myositis
  - Metabolic abnormalities
- Pins and needles in the hand may be due to:
  - Neurological problem: cervical spondylosis, carpal tunnel syndrome
  - Metabolic abnormality
- Difficulty in standing up from a squatting position suggests proximal myopathy, which is found in:
  - Muscular disorders
  - Neurological disorders
  - Endocrine disorders: hyperthyroidism, Cushing's syndrome, hypocalcaemia
- A careful history and examination is important
  - A history of exertion (painting and decorating classically causes pain in the shoulder muscles and may cause nerve injury resulting in the sensation of pins and needles)
  - Has the patient been started on any drugs? Statins can cause muscular pains
- Metabolic abnormalities associated with muscular pains include:
  - Hyperglycaemia
  - Uraemia
  - Hypocalcaemia
  - Hypomagnesaemia

Endocrinology and Diabetes: Clinical Cases Uncovered. By R. Ajjan. Published 2009 by Blackwell Publishing, ISBN: 978-1-4051-5726-1

A detailed history of 'pins and needles' to include:
- Recent activity (painting and decorating; see above)
- Does it follow a particular root or nerve distribution? For example, in median nerve lesions sensation in the palmar aspect of lateral 3½ fingers are affected, whereas in ulnar nerve lesions the medial 1½ fingers are affected

There is no previous history of note and she is not on any medications. She tells you that the feeling of 'pins and needles' affects the tips of her fingers and can sometimes be felt around the mouth. Physical examination reveals:
No gross neurological abnormality in her upper limbs: normal power, normal sensation to pinprick and touch, normal reflexes
Positive Trousseau sign
Negative Chvostek's sign

What does this suggest?
The history and the positive Trousseau sign are suggestive of hypocalcaemia.

What test would you request at this stage?
- Calcium profile
- U&Es

Her blood test shows:
Sodium   138 mmol/L
Potassium   3.9 mmol/L
Creatinine   76 µmol/L
Urea   3.8 mmol/L
Calcium   1.84 mmol/L (normal range 2.2–2.6 mmol/L)
AP   640 U/L (normal range 100–300 U/L)

What do these results suggest?
These results suggest that the cause of Ayesha's symptoms is hypocalcaemia.

What would you do next?

- The cause of her hypocalcaemia should be established
- Low calcium and raised AP suggests osteomolacia as the cause
- The following tests should be requested:
  - PTH
  - Vitamin D levels

Her blood tests showed:
PTH　　15.6 pmol/L (normal range 1–6.1 pmol/L)
Vit D₃　8 ng/L (normal range >60 ng/L)

What is the aetiology of this patient's hypocalcaemia?

- This patient's hypocalcaemia is related to vitamin D deficiency
- Vitamin D deficiency is common in Asian individuals due to:
  - Diet: low in vitamin D and calcium
  - Asian women tend to get less exposure to sunlight as the body is covered with clothes
  - However, we should not automatically assume that hypocalcaemia here is simply due to dietary/cultural reasons, particularly in view of the severe disease, and further investigations may be required

Figure 63 is an X-ray of the pelvis/left femur.

What does the X-ray show?

The X-ray shows Looser zone or pseudofracture (right femur), which is pathognomic of osteomalacia.

What other condition would you like to rule out in this patient?

Coeliac disease should be ruled out:

- Antibodies against transglutaminase (tg) should be requested, which are positive in the majority of patients with coeliac disease

Ayesha's tg antibodies are positive and coeliac disease is further confirmed by endoscopy and duodenal biopsy. She is started on vitamin D and calcium supplements (Calcichew D3) and a gluten-free diet.
She continues on treatment and her calcium profile 8 weeks later shows:
Calcium　2.32 mmol/L
PTH　　4.5 pmol/L
AP　　　320 U/L

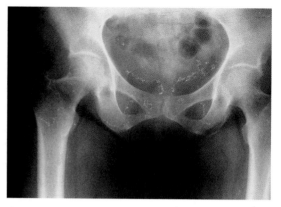

Figure 63

What do these results indicate?

- The tests show normalization of her calcium levels and PTH, with near normal AP
- She should continue on her current treatment and calcium levels should be reassessed in 2–3 months

What is the indication for intravenous calcium administration?

Intravenous calcium should be avoided if possible as extravasation into the interstitium may cause tissue necrosis.

- Definite indication for i.v. calcium:

Box 38　Causes of hypocalcaemia

- Primary hypoparathyroidism
  - Congenital
  - Autoimmune
  - Surgical
  - Radiation-related
- Osteomalacia
  - Vitamin D deficiency
  - Vitamin D resistance
  - Malabsorption
- Hypomagnesaemia
- Acute pancreatitis
- Multiple blood transfusion (complexing of calcium with citrate)
- Increased uptake of calcium into the bone
  - Osteoblastic metastasis (such as prostatic metastasis)
  - Hungry bone syndrome (following parathyroid/thyroid surgery)

- Seizures or tetany in patients with hypocalcaemia
- Cardiac arrhythmias/arrest with associated hypocalcaemia
- Relative indications
  - Severely symptomatic patient

Care should be taken to make the infusion into a large vein to avoid extravasation.

What is a common cause for refractory hypocalcaemia failing to respond to calcium replacement therapy?

- This may be due to magnesium deficiency
- In hypocalcaemic cases, particularly those that are not responding to treatment, magnesium levels should be checked and replacement started as appropriate

CASE REVIEW

Ayesha, a 38-year-old Asian woman, presents with 2 months' history of generalized muscular aches and weakness, and pins and needles in her hands, as well as difficulties in standing up from a squatting position. There is no previous medical history and a detailed history reveals that the sensation of pins and needles can sometimes be felt around the mouth in addition to the finger tips. Her examination shows a positive Trousseau but a negative Chvostek's sign. The history and examination is suggestive of hypocalcaemia, which is confirmed biochemically, together with raised alkaline phosphatase, low vitamin D and raised PTH compatible with a diagnosis of osteomalacia. An X-ray (pelvis and femur) shows changes compatible with Looser zones or pseudofractures, a pathognomic finding in osteomalacia. Although vitamin D-poor diet and lack of sun exposure are common causes of vitamin D deficiency, all individuals should be investigated for coeliac disease, and it turns out that Ayesha has this condition. Treatment of this patient with a gluten-free diet, together with vitamin D and calcium supplements, resulted in resolution of her symptoms and normalization of her abnormal biochemistry.

KEY POINTS

- Osteomalacia, a common condition, occurs as a result of inadequate mineralization of mature bone. Rickets is a similar condition but occurs in the growing skeleton
- Clinical features of osteomalacia include:
  - Bony and muscular aches and pains
  - Fractures
  - Proximal myopathy
  - Symptoms of hypocalcaemia
- Biochemical findings in osteomalacia include:
  - Low vitamin D
  - Low/low-normal calcium
  - Raised alkaline phosphatase
  - Raised PTH
- Causes of low vitamin D levels include:
  - Poor sunlight exposure
  - Poor diet
  - Malabsorption
- Causes of hypocalcaemia include:
  - Primary hypoparathyroidism
  - Osteomalacia
  - Hypomagnesaemia
  - Acute pancreatitis
  - Multiple blood transfusions (complexing of calcium with citrate)
  - Increased uptake of calcium into the bone: osteoblastic metastasis (such as prostatic metastasis); hungry bone syndrome (following parathyroid/thyroid surgery)
- Treatment of osteomalacia includes:
  - Vitamin D and calcium replacement
  - Treat the cause
- Calcium should be given orally and intravenous calcium is only indicated in:
  - Seizures or tetany in patients with hypocalcaemia
  - Cardiac arrhythmias/arrest with associated hypocalcaemia
  - Severe symptoms associated with significant hypocalcaemia

Case 23 A wrist fracture in a 56-year-old woman

Christine, aged 56, suffers a fracture of her wrist after a minor fall. Her past medical history is unremarkable and she is not on any regular medication.

What do you need to rule out in this patient?

As the fracture happened after a minor fall, the possibility of osteoporosis should be ruled out.

What questions would you ask this patient, which may help to diagnose osteoporosis?

- History of previous fractures
- Age at menopause (natural or surgical): earlier age of menopause is more likely to result in premature osteoporosis
- Diet: a low calcium/vitamin D diet predisposes an individual to premature osteoporosis
- Exercise: minimal activity is associated with premature osteoporosis
- Smoking: this predisposes to osteoporosis
- Alcohol: excessive alcohol predisposes to osteoporosis
- A history of steroid use (asthma, inflammatory bowel disease, rheumatoid arthritis): prolonged steroid use results in osteoporosis
- A history of height loss suggests vertebral crush fractures, secondary to osteoporosis
- Previous medical history is important. For example, the following conditions predispose to osteoporosis:
  - Hyperthyroidism
  - Hyperparathyroidism
  - Cushing's syndrome
  - Chronic inflammatory conditions
  - Gastrointestinal disorders

Christine had a premature menopause at 39. Her diet is well balanced but she thinks she has hyperthyroidism due to episodes of anxiety and palpitations. She is a lifelong smoker.

How would this help you in the diagnosis?

She has a number of risk factors for osteoporosis:
- Early menopause
- Smoking
- Possible hyperthyroidism

How can you confirm the presence of osteoporosis?

The most widely used technique is dual energy X-ray absorptiometry (DEXA)
- Two sites are usually examined:
  - Femoral neck
  - Vertebral body
- Results are expressed as T score

Box 39 T score and osteoporosis

- T score below −2.5 is indicative of osteoporosis
- T score between −1.0 and −2.5 is indicative of osteopenia (low bone density but not severe enough to be called osteoporosis)
- T score higher than −1.0 is regarded as normal

The DEXA test shows severe osteoporosis in the femoral neck (T = −4.4) with normal vertebral bone density (T = +1.2).

What would you do?

This discrepancy in bone density may indicate a collapsed fracture of the vertebral body, artificially increasing bone density. Therefore, an X-ray of the back should be performed.

Figure 64 is an X-ray of the back.

Endocrinology and Diabetes: Clinical Cases Uncovered. By R. Ajjan. Published 2009 by Blackwell Publishing, ISBN: 978-1-4051-5726-1

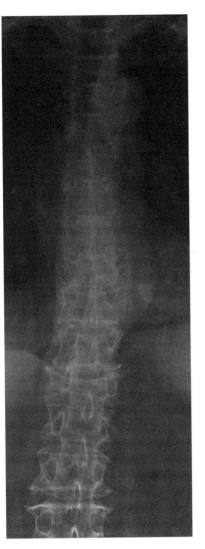

Figure 64

- Hyperparathyroidism
- Growth hormone deficiency
- Gastrointestinal disorders associated with malabsorption
  - Coeliac disease
  - Crohn's disease
- Neoplastic conditions
  - Multiple myeloma
- Inflammatory conditions
  - Rheumatoid arthritis
- Drugs
  - Steroids
  - Heparin
  - Cyclosporine
- Hereditary disorders
  - Osteogenesis imperfecta

What blood tests would you request in this patient?

- FBC: anaemia may be a sign of malabsorption
- Plasma viscosity: raised plasma viscosity is found in multiple myeloma
- U&Es: renal failure may cause osteoporosis
- Calcium profile
- TFTs

Christine's blood tests showed:	
Hb	13.2 g/L
WBC	6.7× 10⁹/L
Plat	330× 10⁹/L
PV	1.71
Sodium	137 mmol/L
Potassium	3.8 mmol/L
Urea	4.1 mmol/L
Creatinine	71 μmol/L
Calcium	2.33 mmol/L
AP	107 U/L
FT4	18.4 pmol/L
TSH	1.1 mIU/L

What does the X-ray show?

The X-ray shows a fracture of the vertebral body, explaining the artificially increased bone density in the back.

What are the causes of osteoporosis?

- Endocrine disorders
  - Hypogonadism: in women, early menopause, anorexia nervosa, athletic amenorrhoea, Turner's syndrome; in men, hypogonadism due to any cause (see Case 9)
  - Cushing's syndrome
  - Hyperthyroidism

What do these results suggest?

All her blood tests are within normal range, suggesting that Christine's osteoporosis is simply due to:
- Premature menopause
- Lifestyle
  - Smoking
  - Alcohol

Her normal TFTs rule out the possibility of hyperthyroidism.

How would you treat this patient?

• In view of her fractures (wrist fracture and vertebral collapse) and the reduced bone density, this patient needs to start treatment for osteoporosis

• Bisphosphonate with vitamin D_3 and calcium supplements remain the mainstay of treatment. Response to treatment should be initially monitored by yearly densitometry

• Other treatments for osteoporosis include:

  ○ Hormone replacement therapy: this is falling out of favour due to increased risk of breast cancer but is still used in younger patients, with a history of early menopause

  ○ Strontium: is effective in treating osteoporosis but can make monitoring the response to treatment problematic (the drug is incorporated into the bone making DEXA scanning difficult to interpret)

  ○ Calcitonin: can be given as injections or intranasally for a short period particularly in the presence of painful vertebral crush fractures

  ○ Calcitriol (vitamin 1, 25 dihydroxycholcalciferol): can be effective but strict monitoring of calcium is required as it may induce hypercalcaemia

  ○ PTH analogue: an effective but expensive treatment and can only be given as injections

---

Box 40 Main side effect of bisphosphonate

• Gastrointestinal disturbances, particularly oesophagitis
• Patients are advised to take the tablet on an empty stomach with a lot of water and should stay upright for at least 2 h after ingestion
• These drugs are usually prescribed once a week together with calcium and vitamin D supplements daily
• Bisphosphonate preparations can be given intravenously, with a newer agent given once a year, thereby simplifying treatment of this condition

---

CASE REVIEW

Christine, a woman in her mid-fifties, suffers a wrist fracture after minor trauma. Due to the circumstances of her fracture (mild trauma), osteoporosis is suspected and a careful history is obtained. Christine has a number of risk factors for osteoporosis including premature menopause, smoking and a history compatible with hyperthyroidism. Her dual energy X-ray absorptiometry (DEXA) shows significant osteoporosis in the femoral neck but an increased bone density in the vertebrae. This discrepancy suggests a vertebral collapse, falsely elevating her vertebral density score, a suspicion confirmed on back X-ray which shows collapsed vertebral body, also known as a crush fracture. Subsequent investigations show normal blood tests and the possibility of hyperthyroidism is ruled out. Christine is started on bisphosphonate together with vitamin D and calcium supplements, which remains the first-line treatment for this condition unless contraindicated.

KEY POINTS

- Osteoporosis, a common condition, is associated with both quantitative and qualitative changes in bone structure
- Causes of osteoporosis include:
  - Endocrine disorders: hypogonadism (in women: early menopause, anorexia nervosa, athletic amenorrhoea, Turner's syndrome; in men: hypogonadism due to any cause), Cushing's syndrome, hyperthyroidism, hyperparathyroidism, growth hormone deficiency
  - Gastrointestinal disorders associated with malabsorption
  - Multiple myeloma
  - Inflammatory conditions (rheumatoid arthritis)
  - Drugs: steroids, heparin, cyclosporine
  - Hereditary disorders (osteogenesis imperfecta)
- Clinical presentation
  - The disease is usually clinically silent until the occurrence of a fracture: peripheral fractures (typically after minor trauma) or vertebral fractures (sudden onset back pain and gradual loss of height)
- Diagnosis
  - Bone densitometry
  - Routine investigations should be done to rule out secondary causes of osteoporosis (particularly in the young)
- Treatment of osteoporosis includes:
  - Bisphosphonate with Vitamin D_3 and calcium supplements: first choice
  - Hormone replacement therapy
  - Strontium
  - Calcitonin
  - Calcitriol
  - PTH analogue
- Monitoring response to treatment
  - Regular DEXA scans
  - Occurrence of further fractures

Case 24 A 37-year-old woman with recurrent flushing

Valerie, aged 37, presents with a 2-month history of recurrent flushing. She has also developed a watery diarrhoea over the past 3–4 weeks, opening her bowels up to six times/day.

What else would you like to know?
Main causes of flushing include:
- Menopause
- Pheochromocytoma
- Carcinoid syndrome
- Psychological
  Causes of diarrhoea include:
- Infections and infestations
  - Viruses
  - Bacteria
  - Parasites
  - Fungi (particularly in immunocompromised individuals)
- Malabsorption
  - Coeliac disease
  - Pancreatic disorders (tumours, chronic pancreatitis)
  - Gut resection
  - Inflammatory bowel conditions
- Overflow diarrhoea (which may occur in the presence of constipation, particularly in the elderly)
- Endocrine causes:
  - Neuroendocrine tumours
  - Hyperthyroidism
  - Diabetes complicated by autonomic neuropathy
- Irritable bowel syndrome
  It is important to take a detailed history, concentrating on one symptom at a time.
- Flushing

Endocrinology and Diabetes: Clinical Cases Uncovered. By R. Ajjan. Published 2009 by Blackwell Publishing, ISBN: 978-1-4051-5726-1

- Severity and frequency
- Predisposing factors
- Associated symptoms
- Diarrhoea

Valerie tells you that she can experience flushing up to three times a day and each episode can last from 10–60 min and is associated with redness in the face. These episodes can occur at any time of the day, but particularly after alcohol and Indian food.

What diagnosis would you suspect?
Valerie is describing classical symptoms of carcinoid syndrome including:
- Flushing and redness in the face, particularly after:
  - Alcohol
  - Spicy food
- Diarrhoea

What is the cause of the carcinoid syndrome?
- Carcinoid syndrome is caused by neuroendocrine tumours secreting serotonin and tachykinins leading to the above symptoms. The presence of symptoms usually indicates hepatic metastasis
- Additional symptoms include:
  - Bronchospasms
  - Right ventricular failure (excess serotonin may cause right-sided valvular lesions)
  - Pellagra-like skin lesions (may develop secondary to tryptophan depletion; see below)
- These tumours can secrete a large number of other hormones including:
  - ACTH
  - PTH
- Tumour location

○ The vast majority of these tumours are found in the gastrointestinal tract and they are clinically silent until they metastasize to the liver

○ A minority of these tumours originate in the lung

○ Other organ involvement is very rare

What tests would you do to rule out this condition?

• 24-h urinary 5 hydroxyindole acetic acid (5-HIAA): serotonin is synthesized from 5 hydroxytryptophan and is metabolized to 5-HIAA. Patients should be on a special diet to minimize the possibility of false-positive results. For example, banana and chocolate may increase urinary 5-HIAA

• Plasma chromogranin A: a very sensitive marker of the disease

• Carcinoid syndrome is usually ruled out in patients with normal urinary 5-HIAA and plasma chromogranin A

This patient's biochemical tests are consistent with a diagnosis of carcinoid syndrome.

What would you do next?

The tumour needs to be localized, which can be done by:

• Imaging
  ○ Ultrasound
  ○ CT
  ○ MRI

• Radionucleotide scanning
  ○ Radiolabelled octreotide scan as most of these tumours have octreotide receptors

○ Radiolabelled meta-iodobenzylguanidine (MIBG)

What are the treatment options for carcinoid tumours?

• In localized disease, surgical treatment may be curative

• Somatostatin analogues (octreotide) can be very effective at controlling the patient's symptoms

• Hepatic embolization: usually palliative

• Interferon therapy
  ○ Around half the patients respond to this therapy, but experience with the use of this agent remains limited

• Chemotherapy and radiotherapy only have a transient effect

What is the prognosis of these tumours?

• Survival of patients with no hepatic metastasis for 5 years ranges from 75–90%

• Around a third of patients with hepatic metastasis survive for 5 years

• Liver transplantation increases 5-year survival to two-thirds in patients with hepatic metastasis

• Patients with hepatic metastasis may survive for as long as 20, or even 30, years

What other types of neuroendocrine tumours are there?

These are summarized in Table 39.

What should patients with carcinoid syndrome have before surgery?

Octreotide injections are recommended in the perioperative period to reduce the risk of hypotension and bronchospasm.

PART 2: CASES

Table 39 Neuroendocrine tumour types.

Tumour	Organs involved	Secreted hormone	Main symptom(s)
Insulinoma	Pancreas	Insulin	Hypoglycaemia
Gastrinoma	Pancreas	Gastrin	Severe peptic ulcer disease
	Stomach		
	Intestine		

Continued

Table 39 *Continued*

Tumour	Organs involved	Secreted hormone	Main symptom(s)
Glucagonoma	Pancreas	Glucagon	Characteristic skin rash
			Mucous membrane involvement
			Glucose intolerance
			Diabetes
VIPoma	Pancreas	Vasoactive intestinal peptide (VIP)	Watery diarrhoea
Somatostatinoma	Pancreas	Somatostatin	Glucose intolerance
	Stomach		Diabetes
	Intestine		Diarrhoea

CASE REVIEW

Valerie, who is 37 years old, presents with a short history of flushing and watery diarrhoea. Episodes of flushing can occur up to three times/day and are associated with redness in the face and there seems to be an association with alcohol and spicy food. The history raises the possibility of carcinoid syndrome as a cause for this patient's symptoms.

This suspicion is confirmed by demonstrating raised 24-h urinary 5 hydroxyindole acetic acid (5-HIAA) as well as plasma chromogranin A. Imaging techniques are necessary to localize the tumour and arrange for appropriate treatment.

KEY POINTS

- Carcinoid is a rare neuroendocrine tumour, which should be suspected in individuals with a history of:
  - Flushing: particularly after alcohol or spicy food
  - Diarrhoea
  - Bronchospasms (can be mistaken for asthma)
  - Right-sided heart lesions
- Diagnosis is made by demonstrating:
  - Raised 24-h urinary 5 hydroxyindole acetic acid (5-HIAA)
  - Raised plasma chromogranin A
- Tumour localization is done by:
  - Imaging (ultrasound/CT/MRI)
  - Radionucleotide scanning (octreotide, MIBG)
- Treatment of carcinoid tumours includes:
  - Surgery may be curative in localized disease
  - Somatostatin analogues (octreotide) can be effective at controlling symptoms

- Hepatic embolization: usually palliative
- Immunotherapy: interferon
- Chemotherapy and radiotherapy only have a transient effect
- Prognosis is variable with survival up to 90% for 5 years in those with no hepatic metastasis
- Other neuroendocrine tumours (all exceedingly rare) include:
  - Insulinoma: results in hypoglycaemia
  - Gastrinoma: results in severe peptic ulcer disease
  - Glucagonoma
  - VIPoma
  - Somatostatinoma

Case 25 A 46-year-old man with an abnormal lipid profile

Oliver, aged 46, is found to have an abnormal lipid profile, during routine tests prior to employment abroad.

Total cholesterol (TC)	*6.5 mmol/L*
Low density lipoprotein cholesterol (LDL)	*5.1 mmol/L*
High density lipoprotein cholesterol (HDL)	*0.9 mmol/L*
Triglycerides	*1.4 mmol/L*

The patient is asymptomatic.

What would you do?

This patient has high TC, high LDL, high TG and low HDL.

• High TC and LDL predispose to coronary artery disease
• Low HDL also predisposes to coronary artery disease
• The role of high triglycerides in atherosclerotic disease is less defined but high triglycerides are probably also a risk factor, particularly as they are associated with low HDL
• Very high triglyceride levels can cause pancreatitis

Any associated risk factors should be clarified in this patient, including:
• Diabetes mellitus
• Smoking
• Hypertension
• Previous history of atherothrombotic disease
• Family history of ischaemic heart disease
• Lifestyle issues:
  ○ Obesity
  ○ Lack of exercise
  ○ Alcohol consumption

The patient tells you that:
He smokes 10/day
His father died of myocardial infarction aged 55
He plays football once a week (but not always)
He drinks up to 50 units of alcohol a week
On examination, his weight is 89 kg (BMI 27) and blood pressure is 169/90 mmHg, and urine dipstick shows protein -, RBC -, WBC -, Glu -, Nit -.

What do these results suggest?

The patient has multiple risk factors for coronary artery disease, including:
• Family history
• Smoking
• Overweight
• Little physical activity
• Hypertension
• Excess alcohol

What tests would you request at this stage?

• Fasting glucose to rule out the possibility of diabetes
• TFTs (hypothyroidism is associated with raised cholesterol)
• U&Es (renal disease is associated with lipid abnormalities, usually low HDL and raised triglyceride)
• LFTs (cholestatic disease is associated with raised cholesterol)
• ECG (rule out previous cardiac event or the presence of left ventricular hypertrophy)

Oliver's tests show:

Fasting glucose	*5.1 mmol/L*
FT4	*16.7 pmol/L*
TSH	*1.9 mU/L*

Endocrinology and Diabetes: Clinical Cases Uncovered. By R. Ajjan. Published 2009 by Blackwell Publishing, ISBN: 978-1-4051-5726-1

LFTs	normal
U&Es	normal
ECG	normal

What would you do now?

This patient has multiple risk factors for coronary artery disease and the following issues need to be addressed:

- Dietary advice
  - Reduce fat in the diet
  - Increase fresh fruit and vegetables
  - Reduce alcohol
- Weight control through:
  - Diet
  - Exercise: this can increase HDL levels, thereby offering protection from atherosclerotic disease
- Modification of other risk factors
  - Stop smoking: effective at increasing HDL levels
  - Treat high blood pressure (needs more measurements to confirm)
- Drug therapy

If the above fails to improve the lipid profile, the following medications can be used:

- Statins
  - Inhibit cholesterol synthesis in the liver and are very effective at lowering LDL and proven to reduce the risk of coronary artery disease. Most commonly used are pravastatin, simvastatin, atorvastatin and rosuvastatin
- Ezetimibe
  - Inhibits cholesterol absorption from the gut, usually used as an add-on therapy
- Fibrates
  - Effective at reducing triglycerides and to a lesser extent cholesterol; usually used as second line
- Nicotinic acid
  - Effective at increasing HDL and reducing triglyceride levels
- Bile acid sequestrants
  - Bind to bile acids in the gut inhibiting reabsorp-

> **Box 41 Main side effects of statins**
>
> - Muscle related:
>   - Simple aches and pains
>   - Myositis: diagnosed by symptoms and a significant increase in creatine kinase
> - Rhabdomyolysis: this is very rare
> - Liver related
>   - Deranged LFTs (may need to stop statins)

tion, thereby increasing hepatic cholesterol requirements
  - Very rarely used these days

The decision to start medical treatment for hyperlipidaemia can be guided by special tables and computer programs, that take into account associated risk factors.

Give one renal cause for high cholesterol with normal U&Es

- Nephrotic syndrome can result in hypercholesterolaemia
- Urine dipstick should be performed in all patients with raised cholesterol

Table 40 summarizes the most widely used antihyperlipidaemic agents.

Causes of secondary hyperlipidaemia

These are listed in Table 41.

> Duncan is known to suffer from hypertriglyceridaemia and is not compliant with his fibrates treatment. His last check of his triglycerides was 6 weeks ago, which showed high levels at 18 mmol/L. He presents with severe epigastric abdominal pain.

What is the most likely diagnosis?

The most likely diagnosis is acute pancreatitis secondary to elevated triglyceride levels.

Table 40 Antihyperlipidaemic agents.

Agent	Main use	Side effects
Statins	Raised cholesterol	Myopathy
		Liver abnormalities
Fibrates	Raised triglycerides	Myopathy (especially if used with a statin)
		Liver abnormalities
		Gastrointestinal intolerance
Ezetimibe	Raised cholesterol (usually as an add-on therapy)	Gastrointestinal intolerance
Nicotinic acid	Low HDL	Flushing
		Gastritis

Table 41 Causes of secondary hyperlipidaemia.

Raised cholesterol	Raised triglycerides
Hypothyroidism	Cushing's syndrome
Nephrotic syndrome	Chronic renal failure
Drugs (diuretics, steroids)	Drugs (isotretinoin, steroids, β-blockers)
Poor diet (high in saturated fat)	Poor diet and excess alcohol
Pregnancy	Pregnancy
Cholestatic liver disease	Diabetes and insulin resistance

PART 2: CASES

CASE REVIEW

Oliver, a middle-aged asymptomatic man, was found to have elevated cholesterol (high LDL and low HDL) with normal triglyceride levels during routine tests prior to employment. Both high LDL and low HDL predispose to cardiovascular disease and associated risk factors should be clarified. Other risk factors in this patient include smoking, excess alcohol, obesity, family history of ischaemic heart disease and mild hypertension. Subsequent tests rule out diabetes and secondary causes of hypercholesterolaemia. Lifestyle modifications are important to reduce the risk of cardiovascular disease, which may improve lipid profile and blood pressure. Antihyperlipidaemic agents can be started according to special tables, which offer risk assessment taking into account age, cholesterol levels and associated risk factors.

Duncan is another middle-aged gentleman with known hypertriglyceridaemia treated with fibrates. Unfortunately, he is not compliant with his treatment and a recent check of his triglycerides showed high levels at 18 mmol/L. He presents with severe epigastric abdominal pain, and, given the poorly controlled triglycerides, pancreatitis is suspected, which can be confirmed by measuring plasma amylase levels.

KEY POINTS

- Hyperlipidaemia is a common condition and can be clinically silent until the development of complications
- Individuals with raised cholesterol, particularly in the presence of low HDL, are at risk of cardiovascular disease
- Individuals with raised triglycerides are at additional risk of pancreatitis
- Associated risk factors should be addressed in individuals with raised cholesterol including:
  - Diabetes mellitus
  - Smoking
  - Hypertension
  - Previous history of atherothrombotic disease
  - Family history of cardiovascular disease
  - Lifestyle issues (obesity, lack of exercise, excess alcohol)
- Secondary causes of hyperlipidaemia include:
  - Obstructive liver pathology
  - Nephrotic syndrome
  - Drugs
  - Pregnancy
- Management of hyperlipidaemia
  - Lifestyle changes are important (stop smoking, reduce weight, increase exercise)
- Medical treatment should be started after appropriate risk assessment. Currently used drugs include:
  - Statins: effective at lowering cholesterol and proven to reduce the risk of coronary artery disease
  - Ezetimibe: usually used as an add-on therapy to reduce cholesterol levels
  - Fibrates: effective at reducing triglycerides and to a lesser extent cholesterol
  - Nicotinic acid: effective at increasing HDL and reducing triglycerides

MCQs

There are 30 MCQs, each with five answers/statements. In some cases more than one answer can be correct. You may find some of the questions difficult to answer and this is deliberate in order to give your brain a chance to do some 'detective work', which is an essential component of endocrinology.

> **1** A 45-year-old woman is referred by her GP with a history of tiredness. Her blood tests show FT4 32.3 pmol/L (10.0–25.0) and TSH of 9.1 mIU/L (0.2-5.0). She was admitted to hospital 6 weeks earlier with a chest infection, discharged within 2 days and asked to complete a 5-day course of antibiotics. She was diagnosed with hypothyroidism 5 years earlier and has been on treatment with L-thyroxine 100 mcg/day since. Her TFTs 2 years ago, whilst on treatment with the same dose of L-thyroxine, showed FT4 21.2 pmol/L and TSH 1.8 mIU/L.

The most likely cause for the abnormal thyroid result is:
a. Poor compliance with thyroxine treatment
b. Non-thyroidal illness due to her chest infection
c. Pituitary tumour producing TSH
d. Pituitary thyroid hormone resistance
e. Malabsorption due to the development of coeliac disease

> **2** A 35-year-old woman is referred by her GP with 2 years of amenorrhoea. She has had a long psychiatric history, but is not currently on any antipsychotics. Her past medical history includes autoimmune hypothyroidism and she is overweight with a BMI of 34. Her prolactin is elevated at 1150 mIU/L (normal <600). Her medications include metoclopramide taken when required and L-thyroxine 150 mcg/day. MRI of her pituitary is normal.

The following statements are true except:
a. Normal MRI does not rule out the possibility of a microadenoma
b. Raised prolactin may be due to overtreatment with thyroxine
c. Raised prolactin may be due to treatment with metoclopramide
d. Raised prolactin may be due to polycystic ovary syndrome
e. Pregnancy in this woman should be ruled out as a cause of her raised prolactin

> **3** The following are recognized causes of raised alkaline phosphatase of bony origin.

a. Osteoporosis
b. Coeliac disease
c. Paget's disease
d. Metastatic cancer
e. Renal failure

> **4** A 37-year-old woman underwent total thyroidectomy for localized papillary carcinoma measuring 2 cm in diameter. She presents 1 week later with seizures. Her only treatment is thyroxine 75 mcg/day and BFZ 2.5 mg as required for intermittent peripheral oedema.
> Her blood tests show:
> Hb 13.2, WBC 6.2, Plt 245, Na 136 mmol/L, K 3.7 mmol/L, U 5.4 mmol/L, Cr 100 μmol/L, FT4 10.1 pmol/L, TSH 7.3 mIU/L.

The most likely cause for her seizures is:
a. Hypothyroid encephalopathy due to undertreatment with thyroxine
b. Cerebral metastasis from her thyroid carcinoma
c. Hypocalcaemia due to parathyroid resection during her thyroidectomy

Endocrinology and Diabetes: Clinical Cases Uncovered. By R. Ajjan. Published 2009 by Blackwell Publishing, ISBN: 978-1-4051-5726-1

d. Raised intracranial pressure due to a pituitary adenoma as part of MEN I

e. Hypomagnesaemia secondary to BFZ treatment

---

5 *The following are recognized causes of hypercalcaemia except:*

a. Hyperthyroidism

b. Growth hormone deficiency

c. Thiazide diuretics

d. Vitamin D intoxication

e. Familial hypocalciuric hypercalcaemia (FHH)

---

6 *The following are recognized causes of hyponatraemia except:*

a. Hypothyroidism

b. Treatment with chlorpropamide

c. Hypoadrenalism

d. Chest infection

e. Acromegaly

---

7 *A 37-year-old woman presents with a neck mass that has been growing slowly over the past 2–3 years and it now measures around 2 cm in diameter. On examination, there is a 2-cm swelling in the left side of the neck, slightly irregular, relatively hard and it moves with swallowing. She has no palpable cervical lymph nodes. She is both clinically and biochemically euthyroid.*

The best course of action is:

a. Reassure that this is probably a thyroid cyst that will disappear and arrange to see her again in 2–3 months

b. Arrange for urgent thyroid ultrasound to further characterize the mass

c. Perform a fine needle aspiration of the nodule

d. Arrange for an urgent CT scan of the neck and chest

e. Arrange for an urgent thyroid uptake scan

---

8 *The following are associated with increased plasma renin activity (PRA), except:*

a. Addison's disease

b. Congestive cardiac failure (CCF)

c. Treatment with spironolactone

d. Conn's syndrome

e. Treatment with angiotensin converting enzyme inhibitors (ACEI)

---

9 *In diabetic ketoacidosis, the following statements are true:*

a. The two main abnormalities are dehydration and acidosis

b. Potassium-containing solutions should be withheld until it is certain that the urine flow is satisfactory

c. Neurological symptoms or signs during treatment of DKA may be due to fluid over-replacement

d. Gastric dilation and gastroparesis are recognized complications

e. All patients with DKA should be covered with antibiotics as infection is a common precipitating cause

---

10 *In non-ketotic hyperosmolar hyperglycaemia, the following statements are true:*

a. Most patients will require antibiotic cover

b. The condition should be aggressively treated with i.v. fluid and high doses of intravenous insulin

c. The prognosis is better than DKA

d. Anticoagulation is contraindicated

e. Acidosis is never seen in these patients

---

11 *In Klinefelter's syndrome, the following statements are true except:*

a. It is the commonest cause of congenital primary hypogonadism affecting 1 : 500 people

b. It can be associated with anosmia

c. Intellectual dysfunction is common

d. It is associated with an increased risk of breast carcinoma

e. It is associated with increased height

12 *A 40-year-old man presents with a 3-month history of weight loss, diarrhoea and reduced libido. His past medical history includes gastro-oesophageal reflux disease and he is currently being treated with omeprazole. His thyroid function shows: FT4 7.2 pmol/L (10–25), TSH 0.82 mU/L (0.2–6.0).*

The next step is:
a. Check thyroid peroxidase (TPO) antibodies
b. Start on L-thyroxine treatment
c. Urgently investigate pituitary function
d. Arrange for an urgent ultrasound of the thyroid
e. Urgently investigate his gastrointestinal system for malabsorption

13 *A 27-year-old man, previously fit and well, developed recurrent headaches for 3 months and a few weeks' history of increased sweating and weight gain. His GP arranged a CT scan of the head, which shows a mass in the pituitary fossa.*

Which of the following conditions is he least likely to have?
a. Visual field defects
b. Hypocalcaemia
c. Hypertension
d. Hyperpigmentation
e. Cranial nerve palsies

14 *Acromegaly is associated with all the following except:*

a. Diabetes or impaired glucose tolerance
b. Hypokalaemia
c. Increased risk of colonic cancers
d. Sleep apnea
e. Carpal tunnel syndrome

15 *The following statements in relation to pheochromocytomas are correct:*

a. May result in hyperglycaemia
b. A hypertensive crisis can be precipitated by abdominal examination
c. Can be extra-adrenal in up to 50% of cases

d. An association with hypercalcaemia usually indicates reduced calcium excretion secondary to high adrenaline levels
e. Once the diagnosis is made, patients should be started on β-blockers to reduce the risk of a hypertensive crisis

16 *The following statements are correct in relation to Turner's syndrome:*

a. The karyotype is XXY
b. Patients should be screened for cardiac complications
c. Most patients are tall
d. It is characterized by high gonadotrophins
e. Osteoporosis is a common complication

17 *Polycystic ovary syndrome (PCOS) is associated with all the following except:*

a. Increased body weight
b. Impaired glucose tolerance and lipid profile
c. Anovulation
d. Reduced sex hormone binding globulin
e. Raised FSH/LH ratio

18 *The following are recognized causes of diabetes except:*

a. Haemochromatosis
b. Cystic fibrosis
c. Chronic alcoholism
d. Conn's syndrome
e. Cushing's syndrome

19 *A 56-year-old gentleman with type 2 diabetes for 6 years is admitted with severe shortness of breath that developed over 12–24 h. His medications include metformin, pioglitazone, simvastatin, ramipril and aspirin, and he has been on this treatment for more than 2 years. There is no history of chest pain. His blood tests show a normal FBC, U&Es and HbA1c of 7.9%.*

The most likely cause for this man's symptoms is:
a. Silent myocardial infarction resulting in left ventricular failure

b. Treatment with metformin resulting in lactic acidosis and compensatory hyperventilation

c. Treatment with pioglitazone resulting in fluid retention

d. Simvastatin-induced rhabdomyolysis with consequent renal failure and metabolic acidosis

e. Ramipril-induced renal dysfunction secondary to renal artery stenosis

---

20 *In gestational diabetes:*

a. The risk of developing diabetes in later life is around 5%

b. Patients with gestational diabetes who require insulin treatment will almost always continue to have diabetes post delivery

c. Congenital abnormalities are more prevalent than in the infants of non-diabetic women

d. Gestational diabetes typically improves in the last 6 weeks of pregnancy

e. Thiazolidinediones are probably safer to use than insulin as they reduce the risk of hypoglycaemia

---

21 *Recognized causes of high anion gap metabolic acidosis include:*

a. Renal failure

b. Addison's disease

c. Cushing's syndrome

d. Salicylate overdose

e. Severe diarrhoea

---

22 *Recognized causes of metabolic alkalosis include:*

a. Treatment with diuretics

b. Conn's syndrome

c. Primary hyperparathyroidism

d. Severe vomiting

e. Medullary thyroid cancer

---

23 *The following abnormality in thyroid function, FT4 31 pmol/L and TSH <0.05 mU/L, can be caused by any of these conditions except:*

a. Thyroid inflammation

b. Pregnancy without concomitant thyroid disease

c. Addison's disease

d. Treatment of cardiac arrhythmias

e. Pituitary adenoma

---

24 *The following abnormality in gonadal function, testosterone 3 nmol/L and LH 0.8 U/L, can be caused by the following conditions:*

a. Haemochromatosis

b. Klinefelter's syndrome

c. Kallman's syndrome

d. Previous radiotherapy for intracranial tumours

e. Testicular trauma

---

25 *In diabetes, the following statements are correct:*

a. Patients with type 2 diabetes never require insulin treatment

b. Maturity Onset Diabetes of the Young (MODY) is an autosomal recessive condition

c. The majority of type 2 diabetes patients die from cardiovascular disease

d. Weight loss is a common symptom of type 1 diabetes

e. Recognized endocrine causes of diabetes include acromegaly and Cushing's syndrome

---

26 *The following are recognized presentations of autonomic neuropathy in patients with diabetes:*

a. Postural hypotension

b. Gustatory sweating (sweating after tasting food)

c. Vomiting and/or diarrhoea

d. Resting tachycardia

e. Foot ulcers

---

27 *The following statements are correct in relation to diabetic nephropathy:*

a. The presence of microalbuminuria is associated with a reduction of cardiovascular risks in patients with diabetes

b. Microalbuminuria can be reversed by the use of calcium channel-blockers

c. The development of diabetic nephropathy protects from diabetic retinopathy

d. False-positive microalbuminuria may occur in the presence of urinary tract infection (UTI) or after exercise

e. Blood pressure improves in the majority after the development of diabetic nephropathy

---

28 *A 27-year-old woman has been complaining of episodes of sweating, tremor and nausea for 6 months, which frequently occur in the morning (before breakfast) and are relieved by eating. Her father, who is diabetic and on metformin treatment, checked her capillary blood sugar during one of these episodes, which was low at 1.8 mmol/L.*

Which of the following are recognized causes for this patient's symptoms:

a. Insulinoma

b. Ingestion of metformin

c. Addison's disease

d. Ingestion of sulphonylurea

e. Hyperthyroidism

---

29 *Which of the following statements regarding obesity are correct?*

a. It is commonly due to a single gene mutation

b. Obese individuals are predisposed to type 1 diabetes

c. Orlistat, sibutramine and rimonabant are agents used for treatment of obesity

d. Obese individuals are at increased risk of both cardiovascular disease and cancers

e. Cushing's syndrome should be excluded in all individuals with a body mass index >30

---

30 *Which of the following statements in relation to hyperlipidaemia are correct?*

a. Secondary causes of raised cholesterol include hypothyroidism and obstructive uropathy

b. CoA reductase inhibitors (statins) are the best agents to lower LDL cholesterol and their use is associated with reduced mortality in high-risk patients, including subjects with diabetes

c. Fibrates are more effective at reducing triglycerides than statins

d. Ezetimibe reduces ileal cholesterol absorption but it is relatively weak when used alone and is best combined with a statin

e. Nicotinic acid is effective at lowering LDL cholesterol and is frequently used as second line in cases of intolerance to statins

EMQs

1 Thyroid

a. Toxic multinodular goitre or solitary toxic nodule
b. Graves' ophthalmopathy
c. Thyroiditis
d. Small pituitary tumours
e. Polycystic ovary syndrome
f. Slow relaxing ankle reflexes
g. Intestinal obstruction
h. High-dose aspirin
i. Hypothyroidism
j. Steroids
k. Lid lag
l. Agranulocytosis
m. Radiation therapy for cancers
n. Graves' disease
o. Osteoporosis

For each of the statements below, choose the most likely answer from the list above. Each answer may be chosen once, more than once or not at all.

1. Serious side effects of antithyroid drugs include
2. Long-term complications of untreated hyperthyroidism include
3. Hypothermia is a complication of
4. Radioactive iodine is the preferred first-line treatment for
5. Smoking may cause deterioration in
6. One type of amiodarone-induced thyrotoxicosis can be treated with
7. Long-term hypothyroidism can be caused by
8. The commonest cause of hyperthyroidism is
9. Thyrotoxicosis with absent uptake of technetium on thyroid scan is diagnostic of
10. A classical sign of hypothyroidism is

2 Reproductive endocrinology

a. Deep venous thrombosis
b. Decreased insulin sensitivity (insulin resistance)
c. Low plasma oestrogen with elevated FSH and LH
d. Amiodarone treatment
e. Low plasma oestrogen and FSH/LH levels
f. Spironolactone
g. Osteoporosis
h. Klinefelter's syndrome
i. Frusemide
j. Addison's disease
k. Premature ovarian failure
l. Increased insulin sensitivity
m. Turner's syndrome
n. ↓ TSH and ↑ FT4 levels
o. Polycystic ovary syndrome

For each of the statements below, choose the most likely answer from the list above. Each answer may be chosen once, more than once or not at all.

1. Polycystic ovary syndrome is commonly associated with
2. Autoimmunity underpins the aetiology of
3. One complication of Turner's syndrome is
4. Elevated LH/FSH ratio can be seen in
5. Pituitary or hypothalamic causes of amenorrhoea are characterized by
6. Use of oral contraceptive pills increases the risk of
7. Menopause is biochemically characterized by
8. XO karyotype is diagnostic of
9. One of the treatment options for polycystic ovary syndrome is
10. In pregnancy, hyperemesis gravidarum can be associated with

Endocrinology and Diabetes: Clinical Cases Uncovered. By R. Ajjan.
Published 2009 by Blackwell Publishing, ISBN: 978-1-4051-5726-1

3 Biochemical abnormalities
a. Growth hormone producing tumours (acromegaly)
b. Primary hypothyroidism
c. Hyponatraemia
d. Primary hypogonadism
e. Osteomalacia
f. Treatment with spironolactone
g. Osteoporosis
h. Paget's disease
i. Treatment with acetozolamide
j. Hyperkalaemia
k. Raised bicarbonate (metabolic alkalosis)
l. Pituitary tumours producing excess prolactin
m. Hypocalcaemia
n. Conn's syndrome
o. Diabetic ketoacidosis

For each of the statements below, choose the most likely answer from the list above. Each answer may be chosen once, more than once or not at all.

1. Hypercalcaemia with an associated pituitary tumour may be caused by
2. A frequent biochemical abnormality in primary hypoadrenalism is
3. Hypokalaemia and raised blood pressure are characteristic features of
4. Very high alkaline phosphatase levels are characteristics of
5. Secondary causes of raised cholesterol include
6. Cushing's syndrome can be associated with the following biochemical abnormality
7. High anion gap metabolic acidosis may be caused by
8. Raised alkaline phosphatase and parathyroid hormone levels are seen in
9. Syndrome of inappropriate antidiuretic hormone secretion is characterized by
10. Early postoperative complications of thyroid surgery include

4 Pituitary
a. Prolactin producing tumours (prolactinoma)
b. Osteoporosis
c. Homonymous hemianopia
d. Metoclopramide
e. Cortisol deficiency
f. Aldosterone
g. Proximal myopathy
h. ACTH producing pituitary tumours (Cushing's disease)
i. Testosterone
j. Bitemporal hemianopia
k. Growth hormone deficiency
l. Dopamine agonists
m. Radiotherapy
n. Surgery (usually transphenoidal)
o. Growth hormone producing pituitary tumours (acromegaly)

For each of the statements below, choose the most likely answer from the list above. Each answer may be chosen once, more than once or not at all.

1. Typical visual field defects with large pituitary tumours
2. Thin skin is a characteristic feature of
3. An increased risk of colonic malignancy has been documented with
4. The commonest functioning pituitary tumours are
5. Prolactinomas are characterized by good response to medical treatment using
6. A known complication of Cushing's disease is
7. Low blood pressure levels in an individual with a large pituitary tumour strongly suggests
8. One hormone that does not require replacement in individuals with complete pituitary failure is
9. A classical clinical sign in individuals with Cushing's syndrome is
10. The best first-line treatment option for non-functioning pituitary tumours is

5 Diabetes mellitus
a. Type 2 diabetes
b. Cardiovascular disease
c. Calcium channel-blockers
d. Hyperosmolar non-ketotic hyperglycaemia
e. Foot ulcers
f. β-blockers
g. Diabetic nephropathy
h. Metformin
i. Type 1 diabetes
j. Heart failure
k. Pain on walking
l. Gliclazide
m. Angiotensin converting enzyme inhibitors or angiotensin receptor blockers
n. Maturity onset diabetes of the young (MODY)

For each of the statements below, choose the most likely answer from the list above. Each answer may be chosen once, more than once or not at all.

1. A strong family history of diabetes at a young age is usually found in diabetic individuals with
2. In addition to osmotic symptoms on presentation, a short history of weight loss is a recognized feature of
3. Obesity is a recognized risk factor for
4. The first-line medical treatment in overweight type 2 diabetes patients is
5. A commonly used medical therapy in diabetes that can result in hypoglycaemia is
6. The majority of type 2 diabetes individuals die of
7. The use of thiazolidinedione (glitazone) in diabetes may result in
8. The first-line antihypertensive agent to use in individuals with diabetes is
9. Peripheral neuropathy increases the risks of
10. Angiotensin receptor blockers can be used for the treatment of

6 Diabetes mellitus

a. Cushing's disease
b. Increased endogenous insulin production
c. Metformin treatment
d. Painful peripheral neuropathy
e. Prevention from pancreatic cancers
f. Severe hypoglycaemia in insulin-treated diabetic individuals
g. Diagnosis of early diabetic nephropathy
h. Glycosylated haemoglobin levels (HbA1c)
i. Diagnosis of type 1 diabetes
j. Exogenous administration of insulin
k. Diagnosis of retinopathy
l. Prevention from diabetic retinopathy, nephropathy and neuropathy
m. Orlistat treatment
n. Urine dipstick for ketonuria
o. Diabetic autonomic neuropathy

For each of the statements below, choose the most likely answer from the list above. Each answer may be chosen once, more than once or not at all.

1. Glucagon injection is an option for
2. Postural hypotension is a classical finding in
3. Testing for GAD antibodies can be used for
4. Secondary causes of diabetes include

5. In a non-diabetic individual, hypoglycaemia in the presence of high insulin but undetectable C peptide plasma levels is suspicious of
6. In a non-diabetic individual, hypoglycaemia in the presence of high insulin and detectable C peptide plasma levels is suspicious of
7. Tight glucose control in diabetes is important for
8. Lactic acidosis is a rare but recognized complication of
9. A test that helps to distinguish between type 1 and type 2 diabetes is
10. Albumin/creatinine ratio is a useful test for

7 Endocrine tests

a. Toxic multinodular goitre or solitary toxic nodule
b. Non-functioning pituitary tumours
c. High plasma calcium and suppressed PTH levels
d. Toxic solitary thyroid adenoma
e. Polycystic ovary syndrome
f. Acromegaly
g. High plasma calcium and elevated PTH levels
h. Klinefelter's syndrome
i. Adrenal function
j. Thyroiditis
k. Conn's syndrome
l. Graves' ophthalmopathy
m. Kallman's syndrome
n. Cushing's syndrome
o. Pituitary function

For each of the statements below, choose the most likely answer from the list above. Each answer may be chosen once, more than once or not at all.

1. Glucagon stimulation and insulin stress test are used to evaluate
2. Short synacthen test is used to assess
3. Raised aldosterone/renin ratio is useful for the diagnosis of
4. Glucose tolerance test is used for the diagnosis of
5. Overnight dexamethasone suppression test is used for the diagnosis of
6. Mildly raised prolactin can be found in
7. In the presence of normal thyroid function, detection of thyroid stimulating hormone antibodies can be useful for the diagnosis of suspected
8. Hypercalcaemia of malignancy is usually characterized by

9. Low testosterone with low FSH and LH levels and associated anosmia are suggestive of
10. Low testosterone with elevated FSH and LH levels are suggestive of

---

8 Medical treatment in diabetes and endocrine disease

a. Polycystic ovary syndrome
b. Graves' ophthalmopathy
c. Painful diabetic peripheral neuropathy
d. Hypercalcaemia of malignancy
e. Hypercholesterolaemia
f. Conn's syndrome
g. Growth hormone secreting pituitary tumours
h. Renal tubular acidosis
i. Hypothyroidism
j. Excess cortisol production by the adrenal glands
k. Pheochromocytomas
l. Gynaecomastia
m. Osteomalacia
n. Hypertriglyceridaemia
o. Syndrome of inappropriate antidiuretic hormone secretion

For each of the statements below, choose the most likely answer from the list above. Each answer may be chosen once, more than once or not at all.

1. Statins are the best agents to treat
2. Fibrates are more effective than statins for the treatment of
3. Somatostatin analogues are frequently used for the treatment of
4. Metyrapone can be used for the treatment of
5. Metformin is a treatment option for
6. Tricyclic antidepressants are a treatment option for
7. Alpha-blockade is a mandatory treatment for
8. Fluid restriction is used in the treatment of
9. Bisphosphonate is a recognized treatment for
10. Vitamin D is used for the treatment of

---

9 Combinations

a. Multiple endocrine neoplasia type I (MEN I)
b. Familial hypocalciuric hypercalcaemia
c. Carcinoid syndrome
d. Syndrome of inappropriate antidiuretic hormone secretion

---

e. Medullary thyroid cancer
f. Glucagonoma
g. Von Hippel-Lindau disease
h. Eating spicy food
i. Ovarian or adrenal virilizing tumours
j. Cushing's syndrome
k. Graves' disease
l. Psychogenic polydipsia
m. Multiple endocrine neoplasia type II (MEN II)
n. Polycystic ovary disease
o. Excessive gastrin secretion (gastrinoma)

For each of the statements below, choose the most likely answer from the list above. Each answer may be chosen once, more than once or not at all.

1. Severe flushing of the face and upper thorax after alcohol may be due to
2. The combination of an insulinoma and hyperparathyroidism should raise suspicion of
3. The combination of pheochromocytoma and retinal hemangioblastoma suggests a diagnosis of
4. Severe peptic ulcer disease that is refractory to standard medical treatment should be investigated for the possibility of
5. The combination of hypercalcaemia and low urinary calcium excretion is suggestive of
6. The combination of rapid weight gain and easy bruising in an individual with newly diagnosed diabetes should raise the suspicion of
7. The combination of medullary thyroid cancer and pheochromocytoma suggests a diagnosis of
8. The combination of a thyroid nodule with raised plasma calcitonin levels suggests a diagnosis of
9. In a euvolemic individual, the combination of hyponatraemia, low plasma osmolarity and high urine osmolarity suggests a diagnosis of
10. The combination of recent hirsutism, deepning of voice and clitoromegaly is suggestive of

10 Miscellaneous

a. Primary hypogonadism
b. Spironolactone
c. Anabolic steroid abuse
d. Vertebral crush fractures
e. HMG-CoA reductase inhibitors (statins)
f. Hirsutism
g. Low dose radioactive iodine
h. Increased lean body mass and decreased fat mass
i. Intra-articular steroid injections of the affected joint
j. Propylthiouracil
k. Renal colic due to calculi
l. Hypoglycaemia
m. Diabetes insipidus
n. Frusemide
o. Immobilization of the affected joint

For each of the statements below, choose the most likely answer from the list above. Each answer may be chosen once, more than once or not at all.

1. Rhabdomyolysis is a rare but recognized complication of treatment with

2. In a muscular body builder, the finding of low testosterone with low normal LH levels is suggestive of

3. Severe liver failure may result in acute

4. In a pregnant woman with Graves' disease, the best treatment option to control thyroid hormone levels is

5. One of the best treatment options for diabetic Charcot's arthropathy is

6. Hyperaldosteronism secondary to bilateral adrenal hyperplasia is best treated medically with

7. A non-diabetic, normocalcaemic individuals with polyuria and polydipsia should be investigated for the possibility of

8. Sudden onset back pain in an individual with known osteoporosis suggests a diagnosis of

9. Growth hormone and testosterone hormone replacement therapy is associated with

10. Late onset congenital adrenal hyperplasia is a recognized cause of

SAQs

Endocrinology and Diabetes: Clinical Cases Uncovered. By R. Ajjan.
Published 2009 by Blackwell Publishing, ISBN: 978-1-4051-5726-1

1 *A 28-year old-woman presents with classical symptoms of hyperthyroidism including tremor, heat intolerance, palpitations, frequent bowel motions, irritability and weight loss.*

a. What clues in the history or examination would point towards a diagnosis of Graves' disease?
b. What are the indications for a thyroid uptake scan in such individuals?

2 *A 41-year-old man has been recently diagnosed with diabetes after a few weeks' history of osmotic symptoms and elevated fasting blood glucose at 15 mmol/L.*

In newly diagnosed diabetes, how can you differentiate type 1 from type 2 diabetes?

3 *A 35-year-old woman presents with visual disturbances. A CT scan of the head reveals a large pituitary tumour compressing the optic chiasm.*

Describe briefly the clinical assessment of this patient.

4 *A 25-year-old is found to be hypertensive at 190/105 mmHg during routine clinical examination while registering with a new doctor. Repeat measurement of blood pressure shows a value of 193/104 mmHg.*

a. What are the endocrine causes of secondary hypertension?
b. When should the diagnosis be suspected?

5 *An overweight 23-year-old woman (BMI 29) presents with 4 months' history of secondary amenorrhoea.*

a. What basic tests would help you to reach a diagnosis?
b. In the presence of hirsutism, what is the commonest diagnosis in this group of patients?

6 *A 51-year-old woman complains of sudden onset severe back pain. An X-ray of the spine shows collapse of one of the lumbar vertebrae and general decrease in bone density is noted, suggesting osteoporosis.*

What are the common causes of early osteoporosis?

7 *A 56-year-old man, who was diagnosed with type 2 diabetes 4 years earlier, is admitted to hospital with sudden onset chest pain and shortness of breath. An ECG shows ST elevation in the anterior leads consistent with a myocardial infarction.*

What is the best strategy to prevent cardiovascular disease in individuals with type 2 diabetes?

8 *A 66-year-old woman is complaining of abdominal pain, constipation and osmotic symptoms. Her fasting glucose and kidney function are normal but her calcium is found to be elevated at 3.05 mmol/L.*

a. What are the causes of hypercalcaemia?
b. In an individual with severe hypercalcaemia, what is the best medical treatment?

9 *A 64-year-old man had undergone a CT scan of the abdomen for suspected abdominal aortic aneurysm. The scan rules out this diagnosis but an incidental finding of a 2-cm adrenal mass is documented.*

a. What endocrine conditions need to be ruled out?

b. What biochemical tests need to be requested?

10 *A 72-year-old man is admitted to hospital with general deterioration and inability to cope at home. His blood tests show low sodium at 117 mmol/L with otherwise normal kidney function. His potassium and calcium are both in the normal range.*

What are the causes of hyponatraemia?

MCQs answers

1. a. This is not an uncommon scenario. Failure to comply with thyroxine replacement results in an increase in TSH levels (loss of negative feedback) associated with low FT4. Patients usually compensate before having their blood test done or before their review at clinic by taking extra tablets of thyroxine, and this results in elevated FT4 without suppression of TSH as levels of the latter require days–weeks to change.

   Non-thyroidal illness, seen in acutely unwell patients, is characterized by low FT4 with inappropriately low/low-normal TSH and can be difficult to distinguish from secondary hypothyroidism. Therefore, checking TFTs in acutely unwell patients should be avoided unless the medical condition is deemed to be thyroid-related.

   A pituitary tumour producing TSH may result in this biochemical abnormality. However, the patient is usually hyperthyroid clinically and this picture does not occur in subjects with known hypothyroidism (as the thyroid is unable to produce thyroid hormones), unless the original diagnosis was incorrect.

   Thyroid hormone resistance is a genetic disease due to mutations in the thyroid hormone receptor and can be divided into:

   ○ Pituitary thyroid hormone resistance: this can produce such a biochemical abnormality due to a compromised feedback mechanism (thyroid hormones are unable to switch off TSH production). The patient is clinically thyrotoxic (peripheral tissue responds normally to the effects of excess thyroid hormones) and there is no history of hypothyroidism

   ○ Total thyroid hormone resistance (both pituitary and peripheral): again this can produce such a biochemical abnormality but the patient is usually clinically hypothyroid (peripheral tissue is not responding to the effects of thyroxine). Normal TFTs 2 years earlier effectively rule out a diagnosis of thyroid hormone resistance as a cause for this patient's symptoms

   ○ Malabsorption may result in increased thyroxine requirement in hypothyroid patients, but FT4 is expected to be low or normal and not elevated. It should be noted that a large number of medications may interfere with thyroxine absorption including commonly used agents such as antacids (Gaviscon) and ferrous sulphate

2. b. A small pituitary microadenoma producing prolactin without detectable radiological abnormalities is always possible (sometimes the tumour is too small to be visualized by MRI).

   Undertreatment with L-thyroxine may result in elevated prolactin due to increased secretion of TRH, which can stimulate prolactin production. Therefore, in subjects with raised prolactin, TFTs should be checked to rule out the possibility of hypothyroidism as a cause for raised prolactin.

   Metoclopramide is a dopamine receptor antagonist and can increase prolactin levels. A large number of agents can modulate plasma prolactin and these are discussed in the clinical section of this book.

   Polycystic ovary disease is a possible diagnosis in this patient, particularly given her weight, which can be associated with mildly raised prolactin levels. Assessing endometrial thickness helps to differentiate between microprolactinoma and PCOS, as the endometrium is thin in the former and thick in the latter.

Endocrinology and Diabetes: Clinical Cases Uncovered. By R. Ajjan. Published 2009 by Blackwell Publishing, ISBN: 978-1-4051-5726-1

Pregnancy should always be excluded as a cause of raised prolactin levels to avoid unnecessary, and often embarrassing, investigations.

3. b, c, d, e. Osteoporosis does not cause elevation of alkaline phosphatase (AP) unless it is complicated by a fracture.

Coeliac disease can result in decreased calcium and vitamin D absorption and, hence, osteomalacia with elevation of AP.

The hallmark of Paget's disease is elevation of AP; clinically silent Paget's disease is often picked up during routine tests that show elevated AP levels.

Metastatic cancers can certainly result in elevated AP through bone destruction.

Renal failure is associated with impaired hydroxylation of vitamin D to its active form, resulting in vitamin D deficiency and consequently raised AP.

4. c. Hypothyroidism does not usually cause seizures, particularly in the presence of relatively mild TFT abnormalities as in this patient. Individuals with severe hypothyroidism, resulting in myxoedema coma, may develop seizures but this is extremely rare.

Cerebral metastasis is a possibility but the original tumour is small and it appears to be localized, and, therefore, distant metastases are unlikely.

Hypocalcaemia post thyroid surgery is a recognized complication and it is the most likely diagnosis here.

This patient does not have MEN I, which is associated with medullary and not papillary thyroid cancers.

Severe hypomagnesaemia may cause seizures but it is unlikely with intermittent bendrofluazide therapy. Also, severe hypomagnesaemia is expected to result in hypokalaemia, which this patient does not have.

5. b. Hyperthyroidism may cause mild hypercalcaemia by increasing bone resorption.

Growth hormone excess and not deficiency is a cause of hypercalcaemia.

Thiazide diuretics increase renal calcium reabsorption, thereby resulting in hypercalcaemia.

Vitamin D increases calcium absorption from the gut and decreases renal loss.

FHH is associated with raised plasma calcium, and it is a benign condition that does not require any treatment.

6. e. Conditions a, b and d can all cause hyponatraemia due to inappropriate ADH secretion.

Hypoadrenalism results in hyponatraemia through renal salt-wasting (absence of aldosterone).

Acromegaly is not usually associated with hyponatraemia.

7. c. This is a young woman with a mass in the neck, which appears to be thyroid-related (moves with swallowing). It may be a thyroid cyst but even this can be malignant, and, therefore, should be investigated.

An urgent ultrasound can be helpful as there are some ultrasound criteria that make a lesion suspicious (increased vascularity, hypoechoic masses and microcalcification are ultrasound features of malignancy). However, some benign-looking masses on ultrasound may turn out to be malignant.

CT scan of the neck and chest may be useful in subjects with thyroid malignancy to establish the extent of the disease and it is also helpful in those with suspected retrosternal goitres. However, it is unlikely to be that helpful in making the correct diagnosis here.

An uptake scan of the thyroid is helpful in cases of thyrotoxicosis and the presence of thyroid nodule to determine whether the nodule is hot (increased uptake), in which case malignancy risk is negligible, or cold (decreased uptake) in which case the risk of malignancy is significant. An uptake scan is not that helpful in individuals who are euthyroid.

The best test in this patient is fine needle aspiration (FNA) of the thyroid. Those with a benign cytology should have a repeat FNA in 6 months. Those with undetermined or suspicious cytology should undergo surgery. In patients with high clinical suspicion and benign cytology results, it is perhaps safer to ask the surgeon to intervene as thyroid FNA can give false-negative results in 5-8% of cases.

8. d. Addison's disease is associated with raised PRA due to low aldosterone production and hypotension, which stimulate renal renin secretion.

PART 3: SELF-ASSESSMENT

CCF is associated with decreased renal perfusion, and, therefore, increased renin production.

c and e are both associated with increased renin production.

In d, there is independent increased production of aldosterone, which switches off renin production.

9. a, c, d. Patients with DKA are dehydrated due to osmotic diuresis and vomiting. They are acidotic due to an abnormal metabolism of fatty acids giving rise to ketone bodies.

Potassium-containing solutions should not be withheld if the patient has low plasma potassium as severe hypokalaemia can result in cardiac arrhythmias and death. Hypokalaemia complicates treatment of DKA, as correction of acidosis and insulin treatment both lower plasma potassium by shifting this electrolyte from the extracellular to the intracellular compartment.

The development of neurological symptoms during treatment of DKA may be due to cerebral oedema that can arise secondary to over-enthusiastic fluid replacement.

Gastroparesis is a known complication of DKA and should be suspected in individuals who continue vomiting, in which case the insertion of a nasogastric tube may alleviate symptoms.

The majority of DKA cases are not precipitated by infection, and, therefore, routine cover with antibiotics for all patients is not warranted.

10. a. In contrast to DKA, a large proportion of patients with non-ketotic hyperosmolar hyperglycaemia have an infection, and, therefore, cover with antibiotics is advised after appropriate septic screening.

Most of these patients are elderly and frail, and, therefore, aggressive treatment with fluid may push these individuals into heart failure. The safest way to manage the fluid status of these individuals is via the insertion of a central line with regular monitoring of the central venous pressure. Despite very high plasma glucose levels, insulin is required in low concentrations in contrast to DKA patients.

The prognosis is far worse than DKA as mortality can reach 50%, compared to less than 5% for DKA patients.

Anticoagulation is advised for these patients, in the absence of contraindications, as thrombotic complications develop in a large number of individuals.

Acidosis is not a feature of this condition but can be seen secondary to the precipitating condition, such as infection or myocardial infarction.

11. b. Klinefelter's syndrome (KS) is the commonest congenital hypogonadism and is characterized by low testosterone and high gonadotrophins (hypergonadotrophic hypogonadism).

KS is not associated with anosmia, in contrast to Kallman's syndrome which is characterized by low testosterone and low gonadotrophins (hypogonadotrophic hypogonadism).

Intellectual dysfunction is seen in around half of KS patients.

The risk of breast carcinoma is increased in these individuals.

It is associated with increased height due to delayed fusion of bone epiphyses (secondary to low testosterone levels).

12. c. Checking this patient's TPO antibodies is not helpful as his TFT results are not consistent with primary hypothyroidism.

Starting this patient on L-thyroxine may precipitate an adrenal crisis if his cortisol levels are low, which may be lethal.

This patient has low FT4 with inappropriately low-normal TSH, suggesting secondary hypothyroidism. Furthermore, reduced libido suggests reduced androgen levels. Weight loss and diarrhoea may be due to cortisol deficiency. Therefore, urgent investigations of his pituitary function are required including static hormonal tests (prolactin, testosterone, SHBG, FSH and LH) as well as stimulating hormonal tests (glucagon stimulation test or insulin stress test).

Ultrasound of the thyroid has no role here in the management of this patient.

Malabsorption may explain the weight loss and diarrhoea but it offers no explanation for the abnormal thyroid function.

13. b. Visual field defects, classically bitemporal hemianopia, are often associated with large pituitary tumours causing chiasmatic compression.

Hypercalcaemia can be seen in acromegaly, but hypocalcaemia is not a complication of pituitary tumours.

Hypertension may occur in acromegaly or Cushing's disease.

Hyperpigmentation can be seen in Cushing's disease.

Cranial nerve palsies may occur with large pituitary tumours or in those complicated by infarction (pituitary apoplexy).

14. b. Acromegaly can result in impaired glucose tolerance and even frank diabetes.

Hypokalaemia, which may occur in Cushing's disease, is not a recognized complication of acromegaly.

There is an increased risk of colonic cancers in these patients, and, therefore, periodical colonoscopy is advised for those above the age of 50.

Sleep apnea is a known complication of this condition due to soft tissue enlargement.

Carpal tunnel syndrome (CTS) is a known complication of acromegaly. The other endocrine condition that results in CTS is hypothyroidism.

15. a, b. Pheochromocytoma is a very rare cause of diabetes.

Abdominal palpation can occasionally precipitate a hypertensive crisis due to mechanical pressure on the tumour.

Pheochromocytoma is extra-adrenal in only 10% of cases.

An association with hypercalcaemia suggests MEN 2, which includes pheochromocytoma, medullary carcinoma of the thyroid and hyperparathyroidism.

Once the diagnosis is made, patients should be started on an α-blocker before β-blockers can be introduced.

16. b, d, e. The karyotype is XO (XXY is Klinefelter's).

Cardiac complications are not uncommon in Turner's syndrome, including coarctation of the aorta, bicuspid aortic valve, aortic root dilatation and hypertension.

Turner's patients are typically short.

Turner's is due to a primary ovarian defect, and, therefore, gonadotrophin levels are elevated (loss of negative feedback).

Osteoporosis is a common complication due to the loss of protective effects of oestrogen on bones.

17. e. Most subjects with PCOS are overweight.

Impaired glucose metabolism and abnormal lipid profile, secondary to insulin resistance can be found in these subjects.

Chronic anovulation is a key feature of the disease.

Reduced sex hormone binding globulin is related to insulin resistance and it is one of the mechanisms for hirsutism in these individuals as low SHGB results in higher levels of free androgens resulting in hirsutism.

LH/FSH ratio are raised in two-thirds of subjects (not FSH/LH ratio).

18. d. Haemochromatosis results in pancreatic infiltration with iron, consequently leading to pancreatic β-cell failure and diabetes.

Cystic fibrosis also results in pancreatic destruction resulting in the development of diabetes.

Chronic alcoholism may cause recurrent pancreatitis, consequently leading to pancreatic destruction.

High aldosterone secondary to Conn's syndrome is not a recognized cause for diabetes.

Cushing's syndrome may result in diabetes through the diabetogenic action of high steroid levels.

19. a. The development of symptoms over a short period of time suggests an acute or semi-acute event. Individuals with diabetes are at increased risk of myocardial infarction (MI), and silent MI (no chest pain) is commonly seen in this group of patients. Therefore, 'a' is the most likely answer.

Metformin is known to cause lactic acidosis, but this is a very rare complication and it only seems to occur in subjects with renal failure, very severe heart failure or those who have an underlying infection. Therefore, metformin is contraindicated in those with renal disease (usual cut-off is a creatinine >150 μmol/L). It is also contraindicated in those with severe heart failure or advanced liver disease. Lactic acidosis is a possible diagnosis in this patient, particularly if he had an infarct, but it will not be the main cause of his symptoms

Thiazolidinedione, including pioglitazone, treatment is associated with fluid retention and this class of agents may, therefore, precipitate heart failure. However, the symptoms are usually more gradual (weeks to months). Also, pioglitazone treatment was initiated more than 2 years ago, making this treatment as the primary cause of the patient symptoms unlikely. However, pioglitazone treatment may have *contributed* to the symptoms through increased water retention.

Rhabdomyolysis is a very rare complication of statin therapy and can indeed result in renal failure. However, there are associated symptoms (severe muscular pain), making this diagnosis unlikely.

Ramipril can indeed result in deterioration in renal function in those with renal artery stenosis, and this is why U&Es are checked around 1 week after starting angiotensin converting enzyme inhibitors to ensure that renal function is stable. In the current case, U&Es were normal, ruling out the possibility of ACEI-induced renal dysfunction as a cause of this patient's symptoms.

20. c. The risk of future diabetes in individuals with a history of gestational diabetes is around 30%.

Patients with gestational diabetes frequently require treatment with insulin, which is usually stopped after delivery.

Congenital abnormalities in children of mothers with gestational diabetes are more common than normoglycaemic mothers and it is one reason why glycaemic control is kept tight during pregnancy in these individuals.

Gestational diabetes does not improve but usually gets worse in the last 6 weeks due to increasing insulin resistance.

Oral hypoglycaemic agents are usually contraindicated in subjects with gestational diabetes due to fears of teratogenicity. Small studies have used metformin and sulphonylureas for the treatment of these individuals but this is not common practice.

21. a, d. High anion gap metabolic acidosis essentially indicates the presence of an extra acid in the blood that is not normally there. In contrast, normal anion gap metabolic acidosis is characterized by a disturbance in hydrogen and bicarbonate ion without the presence of 'an additional' acid.

Causes of high anion gap metabolic acidosis include:
- Diabetic ketoacidosis
- Renal failure
- Lactic acidosis secondary to: hypoxia, infection, vascular event (such as myocardial infarction), metformin treatment
- Poisoning: salicylate, methanol, ethylene glycol

Causes of normal anion gap metabolic acidosis include:
- Bicarbonate loss through severe diarrhoea
- Renal tubular acidosis
- Addison's disease
- Treatment with acetozolamide

Therefore, acidosis occurs in b and e but it is of normal anion gap.

Cushing's syndrome is characterized by metabolic alkalosis.

22. a, b, d. All diuretics result in metabolic alkalosis except for acetozolamide (used for the treatment of glaucoma and high altitude sickness), which results in metabolic acidosis as above.

Conn's syndrome is classically characterized by hypokalaemic alkalosis.

Primary hyperparathyroidism results in hypercalcaemia without any disturbance in acid-base balance.

Severe vomiting may cause metabolic alkalosis through hydrochloric acid loss.

Medullary thyroid cancers secrete calcitonin, which has no effect on the acid-base balance.

23. e. Thyroid inflammation (thyroiditis) can be viral or immune (bacterial is very rare), and typically results in elevated thyroid hormone levels in the blood due to thyroid destruction and release of thyroid hormones into the blood stream (it is *not* due to excess production). This is usually followed by a period of hypothyroidism, which may last a few weeks to months, after which thyroid function recovers. In autoimmune thyroiditis, thyroid function may not recover resulting in permanent hypothyroidism.

In some cases of pregnancy, as well as trophoblastic tumours, high levels of hCG can stimulate the thyroid gland (hCG has similar structure to TSH) causing a thyrotoxic picture usually associated with severe vomiting (known as hyperemesis gravidarum). Only supportive treatment is needed and antithyroid drugs are not used. This is a self-limiting condition that resolves spontaneously by week 20 of pregnancy.

Addison's disease can be associated with raised TSH levels but not suppressed TSH. The mechanism is not entirely clear but is possibly related to deranged thyroid hormone action and abnormal feedback on pituitary TSH release.

Cardiac arrhythmias are frequently treated with amiodarone, an agent that is loved by cardiologists and loathed by endocrinologists, and this can cause thyroid dysfunction (hypothyroidism in the majority and hyperthyroidism in a minority).

Pituitary adenoma is unlikely to cause such an abnormality in thyroid function. Pituitary tumours may impair TSH production resulting in low FT4 with low or inappropriately normal TSH. In TSH secreting pituitary tumours, both FT4 and TSH are elevated.

24. a, c, d. Low testosterone with low gonadotrophins indicate secondary or tertiary hypogonadism (pituitary or hypothalamic abnormality).

Haemochromatosis can result in iron infiltration of the pituitary, with subsequent secondary hypogonadism. Interestingly, it can also cause primary hypogonadism through testicular iron infiltration.

Klinefelter's syndrome is characterized by raised gonadotrophins as the primary defect is in the testicles (hypergonadotrophic hypogonadism).

Kallman's syndrome, a genetic disorder, is characterized by failure of gonadotrophin secretion and is often associated with anosmia.

Radiotherapy of the head can cause hypothalamic/pituitary damage resulting in secondary hypogonadism, commonly associated with impaired production of other pituitary hormones.

Testicular trauma may cause primary hypogonadism with impaired testosterone production but in this case LH levels are elevated.

25. c, d, e. Patients with type 2 diabetes are initially managed with diet and exercise, with or without oral hypoglycaemic agents. After varying lengths of time, the majority of patients end up on insulin treatment secondary to pancreatic β-cell failure.

Maturity onset diabetes of the young is a monogenic form of diabetes (i.e. caused by a mutation in a single gene) and it is an autosomal dominant not recessive condition.

Cardiovascular disease remains the main cause of mortality in subjects with diabetes, as up to 80% of patients die of this condition.

In addition to osmotic symptoms, type 1 diabetes subjects present with a short history of weight loss.

Recognized endocrine causes of diabetes include:
○ Acromegaly
○ Cushing's syndrome
○ Pheochromocytoma
○ Hyperthyroidism (occurrence of diabetes is rare in this common condition)

26. a, b, c, d. Postural hypotension is a classical presentation of autonomic neuropathy, which results in dizziness and even syncopy, and this typically occurs after standing (patients frequently describe dizzy spells after getting out of bed in the morning).

Gustatory sweating is a known complication of diabetes due to autonomic neuropathy.

Gastrointestinal symptoms due to autonomic neuropathy are common and include dysphagia, delayed gastric emptying, nausea, vomiting, diarrhoea and constipation.

Resting tachycardia and fixed heart rate (loss of sinus arrhythmia) can also be related to autonomic neuropathy.

Foot ulcers are usually caused by peripheral neuropathy and loss of sensation in the feet. It should be noted that autonomic neuropathy contributes to foot ulcers through absent sweating, making the feet dry and susceptible to ulceration.

Other manifestations of autonomic neuropathy include:
○ Urinary retention
○ Absent sweating
○ Impotence
○ Defective pupillary reflexes

27. d. The presence of microalbuminuria significantly increases the risk of cardiovascular disease. Therefore, these patients should have aggressive management of their cardiovascular risk factors.

Calcium channel-blockers do not generally affect microalbuminuria, which can be reversed by ACEI or ARB, and in some cases a combination of the two agents is used.

Diabetic nephropathy is usually associated with diabetic retinopathy. In fact, microvascular complications frequently present together, and, therefore, any patient with one microvascular condition should be carefully examined for other microvascular disease.

UTI should be ruled out in any individuals who have a positive microalbuminuria result. Patients are advised to have the urine collection first thing in the morning as exercise can cause microalbuminuria in the absence of renal disease. Other causes for false-positive microalbuminuria include menstruation, pregnancy, any febrile illness and congestive cardiac failure.

Blood pressure control tends to worsen after the development of diabetic nephropathy, and this further results in worsening in renal function creating a vicious cycle. Therefore, tight blood pressure control in individuals with diabetic nephropathy is of paramount importance to avoid further deterioration of renal function.

28. a, c, d. Insulinoma typically presents with episodes of hypoglycaemia, particularly after prolonged fasting. Patients usually put on weight as they frequently snack to avoid hypoglycaemic attacks.

Mode of action of metformin includes inhibition of glucose release from the liver, interference with gut glucose absorption, in addition to a mild insulin sensitizing effect. Therefore, it is not usually associated with hypoglycaemia as it does not result in increased insulin production.

Addison's disease is a recognized cause of hypoglycaemia due to the absence of corticosteroids.

Agents in the sulphonylurea group increase insulin production by pancreatic β-cells, and, therefore, can result in hypoglycaemia.

Hyperthyroidism can result in hyper- not hypoglycaemia.

29. c, d. Obesity may be due to single gene mutations (such as mutation in leptin or its receptor), but these cases are very rare. The main cause of obesity is related to the lifestyle: too little exercise and too much food.

Obesity predisposes to type 2 but not type 1 diabetes.

Medical treatment of obesity includes orlistat, which acts locally in the gut by inhibiting lipase activity, thereby reducing fat absorption. Sibutramine is a centrally acting appetite suppressant but its use in diabetes is not widespread as it may result in the development of hypertension. Rimonabant is a cannabinoid receptor-blocker, which results in decreased appetite and a feeling of satiety after a meal. This latter agent is very effective at reducing weight but is associated with the development of depression in around one in seven patients.

The risk of cardiovascular disease, cancers and respiratory conditions is increased in obese individuals.

Obese patients should only be investigated for Cushing's syndrome in the presence of strong clinical suspicion of this condition.

30. b, c, d. Obstructive uropathy does not cause raised cholesterol. Causes of secondary hyperlipidaemia include hypothyroidism, obstructive liver disease and nephrotic syndrome.

Statins have revolutionized treatment of cardiovascular disease and they are used for both primary and secondary prevention.

Fibrates are used first line in individuals with elevated triglycerides and can be combined with a statin in individuals with combined hyperlipidaemia.

The efficacy of ezetemibe is modest when used alone and best effects are seen when combined with a statin.

Nicotinic acid is the best agent at raising HDL levels, but it is not effective at reducing LDL.

EMQs answers

1
1. l
2. o
3. i
4. a
5. b
6. j
7. m
8. n
9. c
10. f

2
1. b
2. k
3. g
4. o
5. e
6. a
7. c
8. m
9. f
10. n

3
1. a
2. j
3. n
4. h
5. b
6. k
7. o
8. e
9. c
10. m

4
1. j
2. h
3. o
4. a
5. l
6. b
7. e
8. f
9. g
10. n

5
1. n
2. i
3. a
4. h
5. l
6. b
7. j
8. m
9. e
10. g

6
1. f
2. o
3. i
4. a
5. j
6. b
7. l
8. c
9. n
10. g

7
1. o
2. i
3. k
4. f
5. n
6. b, e
7. l
8. c
9. m
10. h

8
1. e
2. n
3. g
4. j
5. a
6. c
7. k
8. o
9. d
10. m

9
1. c
2. a
3. g
4. o
5. b
6. j
7. m
8. e
9. d
10. i

Endocrinology and Diabetes: Clinical Cases Uncovered. By R. Ajjan.
Published 2009 by Blackwell Publishing, ISBN: 978-1-4051-5726-1

10
1. e
2. c
3. l
4. j
5. o
6. b
7. m
8. d
9. h
10. f

SAQs answers

1

a. Important clues for the diagnosis of Graves' disease include: a personal or family history of autoimmunity, the presence of a diffuse, symmetrical and smooth goitre, and the presence of extrathyroidal manifestation of the disease including Graves' ophthalmopathy (GO), pretibial myxoedema (usually in combination with GO) or thyroid acropachy (rare).

b. Thyroid uptake scan in thyrotoxicosis can be requested in suspicion of thyroiditis, thyroid nodule(s) [hot nodule (increased uptake) is very rarely malignant whereas a cold nodule on a background of Graves' disease carries a significant risk of malignancy], and unclear cases (thyrotoxicosis in the absence of a goitre).

2

Important indicators of type 1 diabetes (T1DM) are: young age at diagnosis (but T1DM may occur at any age), absence of obesity (but T1DM may occur in obese individuals), personal or family history of autoimmunity, short history of symptoms (days–few weeks), history of weight loss, and presence of ketones on urine dipstick. Autoantibody tests can be useful in difficult cases, but can be false-negative in up to 20% of T1DM individuals.

3

Examine visual fields for defects and request formal visual field testing. Establish in the history any symptoms of hormonal excess in case the tumour is functional, e.g. prolactin: galactorrhoea; growth hormone: changing glove and shoe size, headaches, increased sweating; and steroids: increase in weight, easy bruising, proximal myopathy. Establish any symptoms of pituitary hormone deficiency, which may occur in large functional or non-functional tumours (pressure effects on normal pituitary tissue), e.g. thyroid: tiredness, dry skin, cold intolerance; adrenal: tiredness, weight loss, gastrointestinal symptoms, low blood pressure; and sex hormones: reduced libido, sexual dysfunction in men, menstrual abnormalities in women. Fully examine the patient for signs of excess or reduced hormonal secretion (see section on pituitary tumours and pituitary failure).

4

a. Endocrine causes of hypertension include: Cushing's syndrome, acromegaly, Conn's syndrome, pheochromocytoma and renal artery stenosis (consequently resulting in increased renin and aldosterone production).

b. Diagnosis should be suspected in those with: hypertension at a young age, severe and resistant hypertension and the presence of symptoms and/or signs suggestive of a secondary pathology.

5

a. Pregnancy test, prolactin, sex hormone levels: oestradiol, testosterone, SHBG, FSH and LH, and pelvic ultrasound, which is helpful to establish ovarian and endometrial pathology and endometrial thickness.

b. The commonest diagnosis in a non-pregnant young overweight woman with hirsutism and secondary amenorrhoea is polycystic ovary syndrome. It should be stressed that taking a proper history before requesting the blood tests is extremely important to establish the correct diagnosis.

6

Gonadal abnormalities, premature menopause or prolonged amenorrhoea or hypogonadism in men. Endocrine disease: Cushing's syndrome,

Endocrinology and Diabetes: Clinical Cases Uncovered. By R. Ajjan. Published 2009 by Blackwell Publishing, ISBN: 978-1-4051-5726-1

hyperparathyroidism, untreated hyperthyroidism and growth hormone deficiency. Gastrointestinal conditions: inflammatory bowel disease and malabsorption due to any cause (for example coeliac disease). Neoplastic disease: multiple myeloma. Chronic inflammatory conditions: rheumatoid arthritis. Long-term steroid use.

7

The risk of myocardial infarction (MI) in a diabetic individual with no known cardiovascular disease is similar to that of a non-diabetic with a previous MI.

It is important to treat a cluster of risk factors in these individuals in order to reduce the risk of future ischemic events:

• Hyperglycaemia, hypoglycaemic agents (oral or insulin) to optimize glycaemic control
• Dyslipidaemia, cholesterol-lowering agents (usually HMG-CoA reductase inhibitors, statins are used)
• Hypertension, antihypertensive medication (tight blood pressure control is important in diabetic individuals). First-line agents are angiotensin converting enzyme inhibitors (ACEI) and angiotensin receptor blockers (ARB)
• Increased urinary albumin excretion (usually measured using albumin/creatinine ratio): agents used are ACEI and ARB
• Increased coagulation: antiplatelet agents, usually aspirin, are given to high-risk individuals, although recent evidence questions the efficacy of aspirin in diabetes subjects
• Increased weight: diet and exercise are an important part of treatment and in difficult cases weight-reducing agents, and even surgery, can be used

8

a. Hyperparathyroidism, malignancy, familial hypocalciuric hypercalcaemia, granulomatous disease (sarcoidosis), vitamin D intoxication, thiazide diuretics, hyperthyroidism, Addison's disease.
b. Patients with severe hypercalcaemia should be rehydrated first and can then be treated with intravenous bisphosphonates.

Other treatment options for resistant hypercalcaemia include calcitonin and high-dose steroids.

9

a and b. Pheochromocytoma: 24 urine collection for catecholamines (usually 3 collections are required).

Conn's disease: U&Es (to rule out hypokalaemia), aldosterone/renin ratio.

Cushing's syndrome: one or two of the tests below can be requested: overnight or low-dose dexamethasone suppression test, midnight cortisol, 24-h urinary cortisol measurements.

10

The aetiology varies according to the clinical status of the patient.

Hypovolaemic patient (dehydrated)
• Renal salt loss
  • Drugs (diuretics)
  • Renal disease (recovery phase of acute renal failure, relief of bilateral ureteric obstruction, salt wasting nephropathy)
  • Addison's disease
• Gastrointestinal loss
  • Vomiting
  • Diarrhoea
Hypervolaemic patient (excess water)
• Congestive cardiac failure
• Liver failure
• Nephrotic syndrome
• Excess water intake: commonly seen in hospitalized patients, who are given too much intravenous fluid not containing salts (such as 5% dextrose)
Euvolaemic patient
• Syndrome of inappropriate ADH secretion, characterized by low plasma osmolarity and inappropriately high urine osmolarity with increased urinary sodium concentrations. Causes include:
  • Malignancy
  • Respiratory disease (usually chest infections)
  • Central nervous system abnormalities (encephalitis, meningitis, vascular event, head injury)
• Metabolic: hypothyroidism, acute intermittent porphyria
• Drugs: a long list including antiepileptic treatment, chemotherapy agents, antidiabetic medications, psychiatric drugs
  • Idiopathic

Index of cases by diagnosis

Index